NEW HOPE FOR INCURABLE DISEASES

NEW HOPE FOR
INCURABLE DISEASES

E. Cheraskin, M.D., D.M.D.
W. M. Ringsdorf, Jr., D.M.D., M.S.

EXPOSITION PRESS   NEW YORK

First printing, October 1971
Second printing, November 1971
Third printing, December 1971
Fourth printing, January 1972

EXPOSITION PRESS INC.

50 Jericho Turnpike   Jericho, New York 11753

FIRST EDITION

LIBRARY OF CONGRESS CATALOG CARD NUMBER: 79-176384

0-682-47387-1

It is our hope that this book will catalyze interest
in the development of an Institute of Health
where one can learn how to stay well
so that there will be less need for
New Hope for Incurable Diseases.

Contents

Preface

MAN IS BESET by two very different kinds of diseases.

One group may be viewed as *curable*. Within this category, a cure may occur without medical assistance. This is the usual sequence of events in the child with measles. The recovery is prompt, total, and decisive. On the other hand, the cure may require medical attention. This is the situation with a broken leg. But here again, the recovery is generally prompt, total, and decisive.

The other group of diseases must be regarded as *incurable*. This, incidentally, is the larger category. Among these, some seemingly can be controlled successfully. This is the case with cancer surgery. Only the malignant site is excised with the hope that it will not recur. Another large group of problems can be more or less controlled, if not eliminated. Examples are diabetes mellitus and rheumatoid arthritis.

Finally, there are many disorders for which there is no known cure or control. These are the truly incurable diseases which continue to destroy, regardless of all that modern medicine can offer.

The medical literature reports isolated instances of success, either absolute or relative, with regard to some of the incurable diseases. The purpose of this text is to examine some of these *hopes* with the hope that two purposes will be served. First, it is hoped that some of the proposals will be employed in persons suffering with incurable disease. Second, it is the hope that bringing these reports into focus will catalyze interest and effort for additional research so that, possibly, some of these hopes will become part of traditional medical therapy.

Thus, here are some hopes for the incurable!

E. Cheraskin, M.D., D.M.D.
W. M. Ringsdorf, Jr., D.M.D., M.S.

ACKNOWLEDGMENTS

ONLY A VERY FEW of the hopes for the incurable described within these pages have been the product of our own research efforts. Most have come from practitioners and scientists throughout the world. In this book we silently applaud their long and tireless efforts which, in the main, have gone unrecognized.

The writing of a book is no simple task and demands the cooperation of many people. We should like to thank our two secretaries, Mrs. Alda McDowell and Mrs. Clara Benton, for the preparation of countless drafts and for tolerating the many and diverse idiosyncrasies of the authors.

Finally, we should like to pay tribute to the Administration of the University of Alabama in Birmingham Medical Center for providing the atmosphere conducive to research and the genesis of this book. We should, however, point out that the selection and the interpretation of the material in this book is our own and does not necessarily reflect the views of the University of Alabama in Birmingham Medical Center.

Our prime purpose in creating NEW HOPE FOR IN-CURABLE DISEASES is to catalyze much-needed interest in nutrient-disease interrelationships and generate additional research so that these and other hopes may turn into realities. In the final analysis, it is social force which dictates medical change. We hope that NEW HOPE FOR INCURABLE DIS-EASES will contribute in some small way to the vicissitudes of the art and science of medicine.

E. CHERASKIN, M.D., D.M.D.
W. M. RINGSDORF, JR., D.M.D., M.S.

NEW HOPE FOR INCURABLE DISEASES

How Many People Are Sick?

INTRODUCTION

THIS IS NOT an easy question to answer with a high degree of accuracy. First, the scope of the problem depends upon the interpretation of sickness. Second, the number who are ill by any definition is not easy to determine. But figures are available, and it is reasonable to assume that these figures are *underestimates*.

The health of a society is traditionally measured by the death rate of its members. Hence, the simplest data are *mortality* figures. In recent times, the concept of health has undergone considerable modification. There is new interest in the total quality of life and not just the life span. Thus, statistics are also easily obtained for so-called morbidity. In other words, data are available to show the incidence and prevalence of cancer, diabetes, heart disease, arthritis, and blindness, to name a few. But, third, information indicating how many people are just ailing is more limited. Phrased another way, a segment of the population is burdened with insomnia, diarrhea, headaches, nervousness, and so on but have not yet become statistics. These people have not yet developed enough complaints, or the findings about them are not so structured that they fit a precise category which, in traditional medical classification, can be labelled cancer, diabetes, heart disease, or arthritis. Fourth, even among allegedly healthy subjects, there are now several score so-called multiple testing health evaluation programs in operation designed to detect early illness. Finally, one significant measurement of the scope of sickness is the cost of medical care in these United States. These points will be reviewed in this chapter.

DEATH RATES

If one examines the United Nations Demographic Yearbook, 1964-1965, one finds infant mortality ranked by country. This, put simply, tells us the number of infant deaths (under one year of age) per 1000 live births. Does the United States show the *least* infant mortality? No! Sweden comes first with 13.3 deaths per 1000 live births. Is the United States one of the healthier countries? No! Actually, the United States is eighteenth with 24.8 deaths per 1000 live births. We are twice as bad as Sweden (13.3 versus 24.8). We are also lagging behind the Netherlands, Iceland, Norway, Finland, Switzerland, Japan, Australia, Denmark, New Zealand, Czechoslovakia, France, Taiwan, Israel, West Germany, Belgium, and Canada. If we could catch up with the Dutch, we would save 40,000 young lives each year.

What about life expectancy? The United Nations source has published figures about life expectancy at birth. The Netherlands heads the list with 71.4 years. The United States is twenty-first with 66.6 years. Though our gross national product is more than twice as great as theirs, the Dutch have a life expectancy at birth of almost five years more than we have!

It is safe to say that, on the basis of these disconcerting mortality estimates, the United States can do much better.

There is a final fact which may be of interest. Within the Americas (Canada, Costa Rica, El Salvador, Mexico, Nicaragua, Panama, Puerto Rico, United States, Chile, Peru, and Venezuela), the crude death rate (number of deaths per 1000 population) in 1938 for the United States at 10.6 was next to the lowest (Canada 9.7). In 1968 the United States crude death rate at 9.6 is the poorest among the countries mentioned above.

WHAT IS THE SCOPE OF OBVIOUS DISEASE?

According to the United States National Center for Health Statistics (1960-1962), figures are now available regarding a number of killing and crippling diseases. For example, Americans in the age group 45-54 years now show 13.2 per cent with heart disease. These 16,000,000 heart patients are equal to the census of the Southeastern United States. By the time the general population reaches 75+ years, 42.3 per cent have cardiac disease! In effect, in this latter age group, almost every other person has a heart condition! Another revealing fact comes from a report by the American Heart Association which states that, for adults 20 years of age and older, 27,000,000 Americans are living with some form of cardiovascular illness. This then means that one of every eight Americans has heart or blood vessel disease.

The United States National Center for Health Statistics also notes that approximately one of ten Americans at the age of 45-54 has arthritis-rheumatism. This figure rises above one in four in the 75+ age group. Figures are also available for diabetes (ranging as high as 3 to 4 per cent), asthma (about 5 per cent), hearing losses (25 per cent), and visual impairment (17 per cent). As will be pointed out in later chapters, there are many millions with disorders not included in this governmental report.

Perhaps more discouraging than the present state of affairs are the trends. For example, in the July 1962-June 1963 period, there were 183,000,000 persons in the United States with 44.5 per cent showing one or more chronic conditions

(illnesses, diseases, or impairments). In the year July 1966-
June 1967, the population swelled to 192,000,000. The percentage of persons with one or more chronic problems rose to
49.9 or nearly one-half of the total population. Three points
should be emphasized with regard to these data. First, the
population increased during the five years about 5 per cent;
the figures for chronic disease 12 per cent. Obviously the disease problem has truly increased in this short interval. Second,
the present record shows that every other American has one
or more chronic disorders (49.9 per cent)! Third, it should
be emphasized that this is the civilian, noninstitutionalized
population, which means it does not include the significant
segment which is hospitalized, in nursing homes, or in the
military. Finally, it should be re-emphasized for these reasons
and others that these scores are likely underestimates.

Thus far we have alluded to the older generation. Mention
should be made, therefore, that one out of five youngsters
under 17 years of age has one or more chronic conditions.
Over a five-year period this figure has climbed to almost one
in four. Hence, it is clear that we are not simply dealing with
an inevitable aging problem. This same trend was noted for
those 17-24 years of age, 25-44, and in the older age groups
under 75 years.

THE NONSPECIFIC AILING GROUP

The simple fact is that one does not go to bed well and
awaken the next morning with a chronic disease (cancer,
heart disease, etc.). In other words, the *final* diagnosis of a
disease is preceded by an incubation period, in some cases of
many years duration. It is during this time that the patient
begins to notice the appearance of various symptoms and
signs. Many are nonspecific and may occur during the devel-

opment of a variety of diseases. Classical examples include insomnia, fatigue, nervousness, and loss of appetite.

Quantitative information of this type is very limited. As an example, it might be interesting to point out observations in members of the health professions (physicians and dentists).

There is a multiple testing program being conducted at the annual convention of the American Medical Association. The program is a very simple one which includes a short questionnaire, a battery of biochemical tests, and an electrocardiogram. The evidence derived indicates that about one in three physicians has an elevated blood cholesterol level (serum cholesterol is considered to be a predictor of heart disease). Approximately one out of three medical doctors has a high uric acid level (which is a biochemical reflector of gout). Roughly one in five shows an elevated blood glucose (associated with diabetes and many other disorders). And so on. These high figures are noteworthy for a number of reasons. First, it should be pointed out that it is usually the relatively *young* and *healthy* doctors who participate in these health projects. Thus, the figures for doctors overall are even higher. Second, the testing program is very superficial. In other words, it is most likely that, if more tests were done, more problems would be encountered.

We have been conducting a periodic multiple testing program of approximately 600 dentists and their wives in Los Angeles, Columbus (Ohio), and Tampa. These dental families annually complete questionnaires dealing with their general, oral, and psychic condition. Electrocardiograms and a fairly detailed series of biochemical tests are also obtained. What makes the program most unique is that *dietary* analysis is included.

The following are some of the findings. More than four out of ten suffer with hemorrhoids. Almost four in ten admit to overweight (and when one admits it, there is *real* obesity). One in five has already undergone major surgery (presumably for a major reason or else there has been unnecessary cutting). Varicose veins are detected in one out of six. One in every nine suffers with high blood pressure and anemia. Ten per cent have a hernia, and ten per cent have or have had cancer. There are more figures, but these should be enough. What is paramount is the high incidence of problems. What is more significant is that all of this occurs in health-oriented relatively young people (in the early to middle forties) *within the health professions* who are a socio-economically privileged class of people. Would it not be logical to project that the figures are even higher in older, sicker, less educated, and poorer folks?

HEALTH EVALUATION PROGRAMS

It must be admitted that it is difficult to delineate those with illnesses in the incubation period from the healthy. One of the difficulties lies in the fact that no one is perfectly healthy. Fortunately, increasing attention is being given to the study of presumably healthy persons. These ongoing multi-testing programs run the gamut from executive personnel in Philadelphia to longshoremen in San Francisco. The incidence of previously unrecognized significant disease varies widely depending upon the age sample, socioeconomic status, health awareness, and the breadth of the testing techniques used. However, the data show quite clearly that somewhere between 65 and 95 per cent of healthy people are not really healthy. This should come as no surprise to the reader. After all, for example, it is well-known that 95 per cent of Americans have dental decay, which clearly is not a sign of health.

It therefore can be concluded from mortality and morbidity investigations that the majority of Americans have medical problems and a sizable number are afflicted with serious ailments.

DOLLAR COST

In the year 1929, the United States spent three and one-half billion dollars for *all* medical care. This means, in light of the one hundred million Americans living at that time, that the average cost per person per year was 35 dollars, or less than ten cents a day. In 1968-1969 the nation spent fifty billion dollars for two hundred million people. This means 250 dollars per person per annum, or 68 cents daily for every man, woman, and child. For 1970 the cost of medical care reached 61 billion dollars. This is five times the 1950 cost and fifteen times that of 1930.

The immediate impulse is to blame this increase on inflation. This is not the case. Actually, only a third of these costs are due to the loss of the purchasing power of the dollar. Another third is due to the rising cost of conducting medical business (for example, orderlies and nurses are paid more). The remaining third is the result of a *true* increment in services such as x-ray, laboratories, etc.

There is a second approach to the economics of the medical problem. What fraction of our national effort, gross national product, goes into medical care? Back in 1929, medical expenditures usurped 3.6 cents out of every dollar we earned. In 1968-1969 the figure had ballooned to 6 cents. The most up-to-date projection is that 7 per cent of the gross national product will be swallowed up by medical expenditures.

There is still a third approach to the problem. In 1929, taxes paid for 13 per cent of medical costs in the United States. Today it is 40 per cent; a greater than threefold increase.

Fourth, there are significant hospital figures. For instance, in New York, Blue Cross reimburses hospitals for the real cost of care. In 1965, hospital costs were rising at the rate of 8 to 9 per cent per year. This was *twice* as fast as the rise in the cost of living. In 1963, hospital costs were projected to double in eight years. For example, hospitals like the Cornell Medical Center were charging about 60 dollars per day. It was therefore estimated that in eight years (1971) the daily costs would climb to 120 dollars. Actually, the projections were wrong. The rise has been greater than expected. For example, hospitals in 1970 charged 100 dollars a day. The compounded rate of increase in 1968 was 15 per cent. If this trend continues, it means that hospital costs will double in five instead of eight years. This being the case, daily hospital rates should be 200 dollars a day in 1973 and 400 dollars per day in 1978. At that time, a six-week heart attack will cost, for hospital care alone, almost 17,000 dollars! According to American Medical News, hospital costs in the major urban areas could reach 1,000 dollars per day within ten years.

DISABILITY INDICES

The total amount of illness in a population can be measured in many ways and for many different reasons. One of the most helpful techniques is the amount of disability a population suffers during a given period. This concept provides some expression of the cost of ill health in economic terms and personal suffering. The most common parameter is the number of days of restricted activity.

In the year 1964, the civilian and noninstitutionalized population of the United States experienced more than three billion days of restricted activity due to illness or injury. This means 16 days for each American man, woman, and child.

Included in the more than three billion days of restricted activity are one billion days of confinement in bed, 385 million days lost from work, and more than 200 million days absent from school. In that year, there were 844 million visits to physicians, 294 million dental appointments, and more than 23 million admissions and discharges from general hospitals. On the average, each American saw a physician and dentist 4.5 and 1.6 times, respectively.

In 1964, about 128 people out of every thousand were admitted to and discharged from average hospitals. Eighty per cent of visits to physicians were for diagnosis and treatment. Four per cent were for pre- and postnatal care. Eight per cent for so-called general checkups. Finally, 5 per cent for preventative services like immunizations.

SUMMARY

How can one measure the health status of the nation? This is not an easy question, and there is no ready answer. At this time, the annual United States investment in medical care is sixty-one billion dollars. This is about 7 per cent of the gross national product. How does one determine whether the investment pays off?

This question has been of cardinal concern to public health officials for a long time. This problem led to the birth of the National Health Survey in 1956. This project is two-pronged. In one, information is collected by interviews. Approximately 42,000 interviews have been performed annually since the inception of the program. Today, information is available on 313,000 interviews which embrace about one million people. The second aspect of the National Health Survey is direct physical examination. The first run in 1962 involved 6,672 people representative of the population from 18 to 79. The second cycle involved 7,000 children aged 6 to 11. A third project is designed to study the teenager 12 through 17.

All of the evidence from the National Health Survey multiple testing programs suggests that chronic disease is rampant in the United States today and that there is a true increase now and a greater increment projected for the years to come.

With a problem of such magnitude, it is fair to ask, "What makes people sick?" This will be the subject of the next chapter.

References

1. American Heart Association, 44 East 23rd Street, New York, New York. *Heart facts.* PR-33, 1970.
2. Golenpaul, D. *Information please almanac, atlas and yearbook.* 1970. 24th edition. New York, New York.
3. Lindner, F. E. *The health of the American people.* Scientific American 214: #6, 21-29, June 1966.
4. Medicine's Week, *$1,000-a-day hospital rooms seen.* American Medical News, 4 May 1970.
5. National Center for Health Statistics. Current estimates from *The health interview survey.* Series 10, numbers 5, 13, 25, 37, 43, January 1964-January 1968. Washington, D.C., United States Government Printing Office.
6. Twaddle, A. C. *Aging, population growth and chronic illness: a projection, United States 1960-1985.* Journal of Chronic Diseases 21: #6, 417-422, October 1968.
7. Ubell, E. *Too much too late.* Prevention 21: #9, 57-63, September 1969.

2

What Makes People Sick?

INTRODUCTION

WE HAVE JUST been told in Chapter One that many adult Americans are afflicted by chronic disease. The singular statistic seldom cited is that, in the final analysis, one out of one eventually dies! This is not of concern here. What is frustrating is that most adult Americans living today in the United States are agonized with one or another infirmity which, according to the best medical scholars, is incurable!

Just sheer common sense would dictate that, for every *effect,* there must be a *cause.* Hence, it follows that incurable disease, as an *effect,* must have a *cause!*

Thus, it is imperative that we grapple with the question, "What *causes* disease?" There are many avenues of approach to an answer. Perhaps the best source is the man in the street, for two reasons. First, he reflects modern medical opinion. Second, as a non-expert, he does not suffer with the near-sightedness which commonly besets those of us professionally involved with medicine.

And so we confront the layman with the question, "What makes disease?" The answer, with surprising regularity, is that man's ills stem from the external world. Take, for example, such oft-heard clichés as "I caught a cold," or "Flu is going around in the neighborhood," or "He contracted tuberculosis." It is not mere whimsy that man's ills are blamed on the world about him; his successes and accomplishments he attributes to his own deeds. Where and why did man inherit such a philosophy? There are two very good reasons. First, castigating the external world for his misery relieves him of responsibility. Thus, disease is no longer man's inherent weakness. Second, there is historic medical precedence for such thinking.

BEFORE THE GERM THEORY

In the beginning, health and disease were acknowledged to be God-given. When man sinned, he was cursed with disease. When he behaved, he remained unscathed. Life and death were intimately tied to religious beliefs.

However, with the advent of scientific medicine, the explanation slowly changed. Increasingly more attention was directed *within* the body as the root of disease. In other words, the body was viewed as the "soil" in which disease occurs. While most of the ancient theories have now been discredited, the denominator which has persisted (even to this day) is that the *internal* world of man is intimately associated with his disorders.

THE GERM THEORY

For approximately twenty-five hundred years, medicine has been probing for the roots of disease. Until the advent of bacteriology, disease was ascribed to a turbulence in man's *internal* environment. Then came Pasteur and his colleagues and the birth of the germ theory. This neat and simple concept suggested that germs are seeds which beget disease. The proposition had its problems gaining acceptance, but it won out finally because it was simple, effective, and comfortable. Now man could blame the cosmos and so regard his infirmities as part of destiny.

BEYOND THE GERM THEORY

There is no question that germs are involved in many illnesses. However, the mere microbial involvement does not willy-nilly argue that the germ is the mainspring. Moreover, the germ theory does not resolve the many contradictions found in nature. Why, for example, can two seemingly similar souls breathe the very same germs at precisely the same time and only one "catches a cold"? There are paradoxes in the field of microbial diseases where it is clear that microorganisms play a role. But, more importantly, how does one explain the rising problems of chronic disease where bacteriology plays less of a role? What is the cause of arteriosclerosis (hardening of the arteries) and rheumatoid arthritis (rheumatism)?

These and many other enigmas now lead us to a theory of disease beyond the germ hypothesis. As a matter of fact, the modern interpretation of disease is a union of the before-the-germ-theory and the germ-theory. It recognizes that disease, gauged by symptoms and signs, is the end-result of an environmental challenge. The peripheral threat may be microbial but it may also be physical, chemical or psychic. In this connection, the new philosophy concedes the importance of the world about man but enlarges the scope of challenges. Hence, the present concept of disease incorporates the germ theory. At the same time, the modern theory of illness appreciates the fact that the capacity of the person to withstand the external bombardment of disease is an equally vital ingredient. This latter factor is cloaked in such terms as host resistance, host susceptibility, tissue tolerance, constitution, or predisposition. In other words, the testimony is now clear that disease is of a multifactorial nature. This means that more than one element operates in the genesis of sickness.

It follows, therefore, that disease may be aborted by eliminating any one or a combination of the contributing variables.

There is sound historic support for a multicausal explanation for illness. In the case of diphtheria, for example, there are two possible solutions. If it were feasible to rid the world of the diphtheritic organism, there would obviously be no diphtheria. One could wipe out the disease completely and forever. Unfortunately, as history has demonstrated, this is impossible. The alternative is to heighten host resistance, or minimize susceptibility, in such a manner that the very same microbe no longer creates the disease. This is precisely the basis for vaccination. That vaccination has worked is evidenced by the almost total abolition of diphtheria.

Vaccination is a workable solution for the acute infectious diseases like diphtheria, whooping cough, measles, smallpox, yellow fever, cholera, and infantile paralysis. However, the chronic disease problems such as cancer, heart disease, arthritis, and others, are more complex. Surely, the environmental factors are not as sharply defined in this group as with the communicable diseases (acute infectious disorders). It follows that greater attention must be given to the individual's constitution in such killing and crippling areas as cancer, heart disease, arthritis, and blindness.

RESISTANCE AND SUSCEPTIBILITY

In one sense, resistance and susceptibility are nothing more than opposites. It really matters little, *descriptively,* whether one succumbs because resistance is lowered or susceptibility is increased. But, viewed *analytically,* there is a big difference. An agent, which when added, increases protection against disease and, when eliminated, diminishes protection, is called a *resistance* factor. For example, Vitamin C safeguards against scurvy; its absence invites scurvy. Hence,

Vitamin C is a resistance factor. Conversely, an agent which when added reduces protection against disease and when avoided increases protection is a *susceptibility* factor. Dietary sugar is not good for the diabetic patient. Abstinence is helpful. Hence, according to the above definition, sugar may be viewed as a susceptibility factor. We shall learn in later chapters that certain foods may serve to increase and decrease resistance and susceptibility in some of the incurable diseases.

The name of Pasteur is definitely linked with the germ theory. What is not generally known is that Pasteur recognized the importance of host resistance and susceptibility. Repeatedly, Pasteur expressed the conviction that the *terrain,* as he called it, of the infected individual often determines the course of the infectious process. In a sense, he anticipated George Bernard Shaw's statement, "The characteristic microbe of a disease might be a symptom instead of a cause." For example, he was puzzled by the fact that hens seemed to be immune to anthrax (a disease characterized by hemorrhage and extreme prostration). He was curious as to whether some unique feature of the hen (different from man, who *can* acquire anthrax) might explain the paradox. For one thing, the temperature of the hen is higher than that of man. To test the theory, he inoculated hens with anthrax bacilli and then placed them in a cold bath designed to lower their body temperature (to simulate man's temperature.) Such animals promptly died and the anthrax bugs were found in the blood as well as in many organs. However, hens removed from the icy bath and returned to normal hen temperature recovered miraculously from anthrax. Thus, a mere reduction of a few degrees in body temperature proved to be the difference between resistance and susceptibility to this dreaded malady. This type of information is becoming a new and exciting chapter concerned not with the habits of infective germs, but rather with the capacities of man which regulate the way the body reacts to infection.

There are, to be sure, many obvious and very likely other not-so-obvious factors which constitute the basis for host resistance and susceptibility. Surely, genetics plays a cardinal role. Certainly, hormones are intimately involved in man's constitution. Host state can be radically altered by physical activity and pollution. One area which is receiving increasing attention by scientists and is spilling over into lay thinking is diet and its contribution to health and disease.

DIET AND NUTRITION IN HOST RESISTANCE AND SUSCEPTIBILITY

Words of definition are in order. First, the point must be made that *diet* is what we eat. In contrast, *nutrition* includes the various mechanisms by which man absorbs, transports, and utilizes what he eats for the maintenance of the myriad of life processes. Diet aids in the support of nutrition, but diet is not nutrition. In other words, it is possible to eat well (have a good diet) and still suffer a nutritional imbalance because of difficulties in the absorption, transportation, and/or utilization of foodstuffs.

Second, diet may be viewed in two different ways. There may be the obvious problem of *undernutrition* exemplified by hunger, and in its ultimate form, starvation. This is a *quantitative* problem of whether man is eating enough food. Additionally, there is the *qualitative* aspect concerned not with how *much* but *what* is eaten. It is very possible to eat enough food but the wrong food. This, in contrast to undernutrition, is the realm of *malnutrition*. This subject will be dealt with in some detail in the next chapter.

While the germ theory contributed handsomely to our understanding of disease, the science of diet and nutrition, as well as hormones, suffered considerable neglect. Even in the nineteenth century, much information was available which showed that cretinism and goiter (reflections of low thyroid state) were in some manner related to iodine intake. Regrettably, because of the fashionableness of the germ theory, most scientific authorities at that time attributed hypothyroidism to exogenous toxins (poisons produced by germs). It was this same philosophy that slowed down progress with beri-beri (now known to be due to a lack of the vitamin, thiamin) as well as many other now recognized noninfectious disorders.

The history of nutrition may be grouped into three significant eras. The first, the *naturalistic age* blossomed from about 400 B.C to 1750 A.D. Its major contribution was that a nutrient is essential to life. The *chemicoanalytic era* (from 1750 to 1900) dissected the prevailing unity into four parts and put into perspective the biologic importance of fat, protein, carbohydrates, and minerals. Thus, the major foodstuffs were recognized. Finally, the *biological period,* extending from 1900 to the present, brought attention to the minute fractions, the vitamins and the trace minerals. Perhaps even more important, the emphasis had shifted from the relationship of *specific* nutrients to *specific* disease entities (e.g., scurvy, pellagra, beri-beri) to the *nonspecific* role of the interplay of nutrients in diseases heretofore regarded as nonnutritional in origin.

Today, much data, indeed, are appearing in scientific literature regarding the role of diet and nutrition in infertility, obstetrical complications, congenital defects, mental retardation, psychologic imbalance, oral disease, heart ailments, and cancer. Some of these relationships will be enlarged upon in later chapters.

The one point for sure—eating as an art is indeed very old, but as a science, very young!

SUMMARY

The evidence is in, and has been for a long time, that numerous factors enter into the cause of a particular disease, even in the case of an acute infectious problem. Increasing interest is being generated in the soil (body) versus the seed (germ). The *science* of medicine, if not the *practice* of medicine, now knows some of the ingredients of host state. Included in this group is diet. Precisely the role played by diet depends upon recognition of the fact that *undernutrition* and *malnutrition* are distinct but interdependent entities. In other words, the *importance* of diet is clear. What remains to be clarified is what Americans are eating. This will be the concern of the next chapter.

REFERENCES

1. Calder, R. *Medicine and man.* 1958. London, George Allen and Unwin, Ltd.
2. Cheraskin, E., Ringsdorf, W. M., Jr., and Clark, J. W. *Diet and Disease.* 1968. Emmaus, Pennsylvania, Rodale Books, Inc.
3. Dubos, R. *Mirage of health.* 1959. New York, Harper and Brothers.
4. Dubos, R. *Pasteur and modern science.* 1960. Garden City, Anchor Books, Inc.
5. Galdston, I. *Beyond the germ theory: the role of deprivation and stress in health and disease.* 1954. New York, Health Education Council.
6. Galdston, I. *Medicine in transition.* 1965. Chicago, the University of Chicago Press.
7. Garrison, F. H. *An introduction to the history of medicine.* Fourth edition. 1929. Philadelphia, W. B. Saunders Company.
8. King, L. S. *The growth of medical thought.* 1963. Chicago, The University of Chicago Press.

3

What Does the American Eat?

INTRODUCTION

THE CARDINAL POINT stressed in Chapter One is that practically every other adult American living in the United States today suffers with one or more incurable diseases. Emphasized in Chapter Two is the salient fact that increasing attention is being shifted from the *seed* (the external world, germs) to the *soil* (the internal environment or body) in the causation of disease. The additional thought stressed in the last chapter is that diet plays a role in determining the composition of the soil or, as we put it, the diet is one thread in the fabric of host resistance and susceptibility. It follows, then, that we ought to take a hard look at what the American eats. More importantly, we should ask ourselves the question, "How good or bad is the American diet and what are the reasons for its adequacy or inadequacy?" This will be the substance of this chapter.

WHAT ARE WE EATING?

We are told that we should be eating three squares a day. The fact of the matter is that the typical American eats less than three meals daily. About one out of six persons in the 18-24 year age category omits breakfast. About 8-14 per cent of Americans skip lunch. Approximately one out of nine misses the evening meal. If breakfast is consumed, it usually includes a cup of coffee with sugar and possibly cream plus a pastry or a donut or two. Some time during the midmorning there is a "coffee break" so named because there is generally coffee with sugar and perhaps cream or a soft drink and even a snack, often cookies of some kind. The customary American lunch, if it is not skipped, is a sandwich and a beverage. The sandwich most often consists of a thin slice of meat on white bread. The beverage is coffee, tea with sugar and perhaps cream, or a soft drink. Not infrequently there is some sort of dessert like pie or ice cream. The mid-afternoon break is a carbon copy of the midmorning interlude. Finally, there is the evening meal which usually includes meat, fish, or fowl, vegetables, perhaps a salad, a beverage like coffee or tea or milk and a dessert. This is the popular story of what the typical Amercan consumes during an average day.

HOW GOOD OR BAD IS OUR DIET?

There are two approaches to this question. First, it might be well to analyze Mr. America's diet according to the recommendations set forth by the Food and Nutrition Board of the National Research Council. The Food and Nutrition Board, established in 1940 under the Division of Biology and Agriculture of the National Research Council, is an advisory body in the field of food and nutrition. The members of the Board are appointed from among leaders in the sciences related to food and nutrition on the basis of their qualifications of experience and judgment to deal with the many and diverse problems that arise. The Food and Nutrition Board sponsors needed research and assists in the interpretation of data in the interest of the public welfare.

Since 1940, the Food and Nutrition Board has periodically set formulations for daily nutrient intake judged to be adequate for the maintenance of sound nutrition in the United States. The first edition of Recommended Dietary Allowances (the official edict) was published in 1943. The last revision, the seventh, was released in 1968.

In January 1968, the United States Department of Agriculture published the results of its spring of 1965 nationwide dietary survey. According to their findings, approximately 50 per cent of the 7,500 households surveyed had diets which failed to meet the Recommended Dietary Allowances (referred to as the RDA) for one or more nutrients. Although the dietary patterns were poorer in low-income families, more than one-third of the households with incomes of $10,000 and over reported inadequate diets.

According to the Food and Nutrition Board, the consumption of less than two-thirds of the Recommended Dietary Allowances for any nutrient is viewed as suboptimal. Analyses by the United States Department of Agriculture of the intake of eight nutrients revealed that the percentage of diets providing less than two-thirds of the RDA ranged from one to 13 per cent. Approximately one-fifth of the diets supplied less than two-thirds of the allowances for one or more nutrients. These diets are rated definitely poor.

In brief, the observations of the United States Department of Agriculture and every other similar survey suggests that the American diet leaves much to be desired. In a review of these data, the Council on Foods and Nutrition of the American Medical Association recently reported to the AMA Board of Trustees that both malnutrition and hunger (undernutrition) are evident in America today. They note that although malnutrition is much more prevalent, the classical deficiencies of the underfed—scurvy, beri-beri, pellagra, and rickets—are still evident in alarming proportions. As a result of malnutrition and hunger, the Council points out that man is deprived physically, mentally, and socially. (A recent symposium at the University of Alabama in Birmingham explored "The Role of Malnutrition in the Pathogenesis of Slums"— February 10-11, 1970).

There is a second way of viewing the American diet. What is good and bad about eating habits can be derived from observations in three categories. First, it would be informative to analyze the dietary patterns associated with gross illness. In other words, "What Do Sick People Eat?" Second, it would be equally helpful to study the dietary regimes of those with incipient illness (during the incubation period of disease). Phrased another way, "What are the eating habits of individuals who constantly report many and diverse nonspecific complaints such as recurrent headaches, irritability, insomnia, etc.?" Lastly, it may prove rewarding to ferret out the diet in relatively healthy subjects, individuals without symptoms and signs.

Numerous studies have been reported of the diets of patients with classical, and allegedly nonnutritional problems such as infertility, obstetrical complications, congenital defects, mental retardation, psychologic imbalance, cancer, and heart disease. There are, of course, differences and considerable overlap in the results. However, the common denominators include too much sugar and other highly processed (refined carbohydrate) products, too little protein and especially of the animal (meat, fish, fowl) type, and suboptimal amounts of vitamins and minerals. This, in summary form, is what sick people eat!

Inquiries of the dietary patterns of subjects with incipient illness are much more limited when compared with the observations in individuals with classical disease. Notwithstanding the paucity of data, the evidence suggests that people in the gray area (in the incubation zone) display diets not appreciably different from those with obvious disease. In other words, this group is also characterized by too much sugar and other highly processed (refined carbohydrate) products, too little protein and especially of the animal variety, and not enough vitamins and minerals. This, in brief, is what people with incipient illness eat!

Finally, even fewer analyses have been conducted of the dietary patterns in relatively healthy persons. The available information suggests that such individuals consume relatively little sugar and other highly processed (refined carbohydrate) foodstuffs, much more protein than sick people, and a higher intake of vitamins and minerals. This, based upon available data, is what healthy people eat!

WHY IS THE AMERICAN DIET INADEQUATE?

There are two reasons, *undernutrition* and *malnutrition.* The distinction between these two terms has already been made (Chapter Two).

The problem of *undernutrition* is largely related to economics. It is now abundantly clear that a significant segment of the American public cannot afford to purchase enough food to maintain health and prevent illness. It is assumed in some circles that this is the sole or, at least, the most important problem with respect to nutrition in the United States. This is not true. A much larger segment is suffering with *malnutrition* rather than *undernutrition.* The problem of malnutrition is, in part, a function of poverty. However, the principal determinant is ignorance of what constitutes an optimal diet.

One of the biggest contributors to the inadequacy of the American diet is the change which has occurred in the nutrient content of foodstuffs in recent years. A helpful approach to this point is to review the nutrient alterations which occur from the *garden to the gullet.* In other words, we must ask what effect does soil quality, food species, transportation and storage, purchasing patterns, food preparation techniques, rinsing, defrosting, and other elements exert upon the nutrient content of foods?

With regard to soil quality, it is interesting to report that the nutrient contents of foods grown in the United States have been compared with similar foods randomly chosen from comparatively underdeveloped countries such as Mexico and others in Central America. These investigations demonstrate that, in many instances, foods plucked from Mexican soil, for example, possess higher nutritive value than like foods taken from American earth. Hence, soil quality may conceivably contribute in some small way to the inadequacy of the American diet.

We are told by the Food and Nutrition Board of the National Research Council that we should consume about 60 milligrams of Vitamin C each day. We are led to believe that a tumbler of orange juice contains approximately 60 milligrams. What we have not been told is that different oranges, based upon species, picked at different times of the year can vary as much as fourfold in Vitamin C content. Hence, it is very possible to drink a glass of orange juice each day and still not acquire enough Vitamin C. Thus, food species may possibly contribute in a small measure to the inadequacy of the American diet.

The complex nature of the American society has been amply publicized. What has not been brought home to us is that the complexities of our culture extend to our food quality. For example, foods are grown in one region of the country and must be transported several thousand miles to the consumer in another region. The food must then be stored and held until the price is right to sell. *The evidence is now clear that the transportation and storage of food always leads to a reduction in nutrients.* Hence, here is a third link in the chain which contributes to nutrient loss in the journey from the garden to the gullet.

Because of the complexity of our society, as well as for esthetic reasons, many foodstuffs consumed in the United States are processed. These techniques, almost without exception, lead to a decrease of one or more nutrients. Additionally, many foreign molecules are included as additives for preservation purposes as well as for esthetic reasons. Hence, there is regularly nutrient loss during processing.

The wisdom of the food purchaser is largely determined by advertising policies and techniques, the motivation for which is purely commercial. Little or no consideration is given to the nutrient value of food in the usual forms of commercial advertising. These policies dominate the purchaser, usually the housewife. Generally, such policies do not contribute to the value of foods. Thus, the ignorance of the consumer plays a role in nutrient loss.

Once the food is brought into the home, it undergoes specific types of preparation. For example, many foods are washed. Considerable investigation has indicated that the mere washing of foods produces nutrient loss. The specific amount of different nutrients which are lost vary substantially with the extent and the type of washing as well as the initial nutrient content. However, one can safely say that, with rinsing, there is an across-the-board loss in nutrient value.

It should be evident to the reader that increasingly more frozen foods are purchased. These foodstuffs, before preparation, are defrosted. It is now clear that with this process there is a loss of nutrient value. The precise deficit for a particular nutrient and a special food will vary widely. However, the general statement can be made that, with defrosting, there is nutrient loss.

Sooner or later, many of the foods to be consumed are

cooked. There is an extensive literature on the effect of cooking upon nutrient value. Once again, the figures vary widely with the type of cooking and the specific foodstuff. However, there seems to be general agreement, that there is considerable loss of nutrient value during food preparation. In fact, some nutrients, such as Vitamin C, can vanish completely.

Obviously, what is cooked is intended to be consumed. Precisely how much of the food served is actually eaten has been studied. Surveys have shown that teenagers particularly may not eat the food which the mother prepares. As a matter of fact, it has been said that the poorest diets in the American culture are among the aged and teenagers, particularly in the young female.

Finally, much of our eating is done away from home, usually in restaurants. Here food is necessarily prepared in advance and served during specific hours. Data have been collected, for example, on the Vitamin C content of potatoes at a steam table. The evidence indicates that within one hour practically all of the Vitamin C may have disappeared.

It is clear, from this brief discussion, that as food passes from the garden to the gullet, there is always nutrient loss. It is true that many foods are fortified. However, it is also a fact that the enrichment replaces only a few of the nutrients which have been lost.

SUMMARY

There is reason to believe that two dietary problems exist in the United States. One of these may be regarded as undernutrition which is largely a problem in poor people. The other, malnutrition, occurs in a significant number of households where economics is not a problem.

According to the recent survey of the dietary patterns of

Americans, it is now clear that there is a major deficit in calcium, Vitamin A, Vitamin C, and in the female, iron.

One very important point has to do with sugar and highly processed (refined) carbohydrate products. At the present time, the average American consumes 115 pounds of sugar each year. This, in simple terms, means that each man, woman, and child eats one teaspoonful each hour 365 days a year. Of what significance is this? It is important for three reasons:

1. These foods are poor in protein, vitamin, and mineral content.
2. Their utilization requires large quantities of vitamins and minerals [which have to be stolen from other foods or the body tissues].
3. They replace foods [meat, vegetables, fruits] which are rich in vitamins, minerals, and protein.

This combination of deficits leads to malnutrition rather than undernutrition. As a living example, obesity (overweight) is America's number one nutritional disorder!

The additional problem is that we now live in a culture where decrease in nutrient value occurs as food passes from the garden to the gullet.

In view of what has been said earlier regarding the high incidence of incurable disease added to the fact that diet plays a role in host resistance and compounded now by the problem that the American diet is inadequate, it is now fitting to turn our attention to some of the incurable diseases and see if there is any hope through dietary change.

REFERENCES

1. Cheraskin, E., Ringsdorf, W. M., Jr., and Clark, J. W. *Diet and disease.* 1968. Emmaus, Pennsylvania, Rodale Books, Inc.
2. Clark, J. W., Cheraskin, E., and Ringsdorf, W. M., Jr. *Diet and*

the periodontal patient. 1970. Springfield, Illinois, Charles C. Thomas.

3. Council on Foods and Nutrition of the American Medical Association. *Malnutrition and hunger in the United States.* Journal of The American Medical Association 213: #2, 272-275, July 13, 1970.
4. Food and Nutrition Board. National Research Council. *Recommended dietary allowances.* Publication 1964. Seventh Edition, 1968, Washington, D.C., National Academy of Sciences.
5. Food and Nutrition News, April 1969.
6. Goodhart, R. S. *How well nourished are Americans?* II. National Vitamin Foundation Report for 1961-1963. New York.
7. Harris, R. S., and Loesecke, H. V. *Nutritional Evaluation of Food Processing.* 1960. New York, John Wiley and Sons.
8. United States Department of Agriculture. Agricultural Research Service. *Food consumption of households in the United States. Spring 1965.* Household Food Consumption Survey. Reports 1-5, 1968. Washington, D.C., United States Government Printing Office.
9. *Vitamin defects found in many hospitalized.* Medical Tribune and Medical News 6: #35, 1, 26, 22 March 1965.
10. Yudkin. J. *Patterns and trends in carbohydrate consumption and their relation to disease.* Proceedings of the Nutrition Society 23: #2, 149-162, 1964.

4

Is There Hope for the Patient With Multiple Sclerosis?

INTRODUCTION

FOR ANYONE WITH multiple sclerosis (usually referred to as MS), the answers to these five questions are very important:

What is it?

What causes it?

How common is it?

What cures it?

Is there more hope?

WHAT IS IT?

Multiple sclerosis (MS) is a chronic and often lifelong disease characterized by symptoms and signs indicating the presence of multiple lesions in the white matter of the brain and spinal cord. The lesion (defect) is essentially a demyelinization or destruction of the protective covering (myelin sheath) of the nerves in a nerve tract. This loss of insulation produces a conduction defect so that the nerves work erratically, weakly, or not at all. One might compare this to an electrical short circuit produced by a loss of the protective covering of an electric wire. Naturally, the nature of MS findings in a given case will depend on the location of the diseased nerve tracts. The course of MS is often characterized by relapses of increasing severity and duration, with about 50 per cent of those affected becoming incapacitated within ten years of the onset. Its importance as a cause of disability among young people is indicated by the fact that 71 per cent of the 2,001 workers granted Social Security disability benefits in 1964 from this impairment were under 50 years of age. In contrast, only 14 per cent of 11,368 workers granted such benefits because of strokes (the leading crippler of the nervous system) were under 50.

Authorities now feel that the average duration of life from onset of this disease may be about 27 years.

WHAT CAUSES IT?

Search for an agent which causes MS has taxed the ingenuity of many investigators for decades. Part of the problem may be the fact that MS like all diseases is multifactorial in origin. This point was made in Chapter Two. Little concrete information is available concerning the etiology except that it occurs more often than could be accounted for by chance in more than one family member. This should not necessarily be taken to mean a genetic transmission. It may suggest that common environmental factors and/or an inherited predisposition may make individuals more susceptible or less resistant to the unknown agent or agents responsible for the demyelinating process. It has recently been proposed that infection or an allergy to an infecting organism or a chemical substance foreign to the body may play a role in causing MS.

HOW COMMON IS IT?

The number of persons in the United States afflicted with MS is estimated to range between 70,000 and 250,000. The latter figure probably includes many cases, especially in the early stages, which may not have been diagnosed or reported because of the remittant nature of the disease. Prevalence in northern cities has been found to be substantially higher than in southern communities, ranging from 64 per 100,000 white persons in Rochester, Minnesota, to 13 in New Orleans, Louisiana. The distribution of MS also roughly parallels technologic advancement and sanitary standards of the population. *In other words, the more primitive the society the less the MS problem.*

Northern states are reported to have death rates above the national average of .8 per 100,000 population. States in the southern latitudes have rates below. The rate of 1.4 in Montana, North Dakota, and Nebraska is almost five times greater than in Georgia and Louisiana.

Mortality from MS is largely concentrated in midlife with more than one-half of the deaths occurring between 45 and 65 years of age. With advancing age, the rate per 100,000 population increases from 0.4 at 25-34 years to 2.1 at ages 55-64. Among females, who generally have an earlier onset, peak mortality rates begin ten years earlier. Whites are noted to have twice the rate for nonwhites, with this difference increasing with age. The tendency for females and the white population to seek more and earlier medical care may account for some of these sex and color mortality differences. Mortality statistics are believed to understate the number of persons dying from MS since a considerable number with MS are reported as dying from other causes.

WHAT CURES IT?

According to medical consensus, no prevention, cure, or specific treatment has been found.

Despite the large number of remedies which have been tried, no drug therapy appears to have any influence on the course of the disease [Harrison, et al., *Principles of internal medicine,* 1966].

IS THERE MORE HOPE?

In an exciting preliminary report in *The Journal of the American Medical Association,* Doctor Glen Thomas Sawyer is optimistic! Reading of the beneficial effects of tolbutamide therapy in acne vulgaris (most common form of pimples) prompted this scientist to use the drug in a young multiple sclerosis patient who had severe acne on his back. Not only was there a remarkable improvement in the acne but simultaneously a striking remission of the MS symptoms. Although Doctor Sawyer carefully searched the medical literature, he could find no mention of this treatment.

While designing this preliminary report, Doctor Sawyer elected to evaluate not only the effects of tolbutamide but of dietary carbohydrate intake as well. The latter was included because of the widespread use of tolbutamide in the treatment of mild diabetes mellitus.

The administration of tolbutamide in seven patients (22 to 46 years of age) with neurologic evidence of extensive nerve damage was followed by a definite clinical remission in all cases. In some of the patients this improvement was repeated on several occasions with each drug trial period separated by a period of placebo (blank pill) administration. In other experiments a high carbohydrate diet produced an accentuation of the MS symptoms and signs. Replacement of the high carbohydrate intake with a diabetic (low carbohydrate) diet, however, had the opposite effect—the clinical findings rapidly decreased. Both Doctor Sawyer and the patients became aware of the improvement or worsening of symptoms two to seven days after a change in either drug or diet. Parenthetically, the MS symptoms evaluated were coordination, endurance, spasticity, bladder control, ocular findings, sensory changes and speech.

Doctor Sawyer described the dramatic improvement with tolbutamide alone in one patient like this:

Case 1.—A 22-year-old man, having had symptoms of multiple sclerosis for two years, was almost asymptomatic [without symptoms and signs] seven months prior to admission. His disease began to progress rapidly soon after that time, however, so that on admission, in spite of several 10-day courses of ACTH [this means adrenocorticotrophic hormone which is a pituitary hormone] given intravenously, ataxia [staggering] was so severe that he was just able to transfer between wheel chair and bed. Vertigo [dizziness], diplopia [double vision], and severe numbness of the hands and feet were also constant problems.

Examination revealed severe acne vulgaris [pimples] of the patient's back, impaired conjugate eye movements, bilateral horizontal nystagmus, a left hyperreflexia, sustained ankle clonus bilaterally, hypalgesia bilaterally below the T-6 level, and pronounced bilateral signs of cerebellar dysfunction [all of these are reflections of nerve disease]. All laboratory tests, including spinal fluid examination and an oral glucose tolerance test, gave results that were within normal limits.

The patient received a regular hospital diet and 0.5 Gm. tolbutamide every day for 18 days soon after admission. During this period he showed remarkable improvement so that, toward the end of his stay, he no longer had numbness and was able to walk well with a cane. Vertigo and diplopia, although still present, were much improved.

For the next 10 days a placebo capsule replaced the daily dose of tolbutamide, and he remained on a regular diet. Three days after the placebo capsules were begun he began to notice numbness of the right hand again. Tolbutamide, 0.5 Gm., was given daily for the next 23 days, during which time the numbness again disappeared and the hypesthesia and hypalgesia [reduction in sensation] were no longer demonstrable. At the time of discharge this patient was asymptomatic except for a slight unsteadiness when attempting to walk rapidly. He was entirely free of diplopia and numbness. [Parenthetic statements added].

Three dietary regimes, the regular hospital diet, a high carbohydrate diet and a diabetic diet, were observed by Doctor Sawyer to produce dramatic changes in the MS clinical picture.

APPROXIMATE COMPOSITION OF DIETS:

Regular hospital diet
calories   2,250
   protein   75 gm.
   fat   135 gm.
   carbohydrate   195 gm.

High-carbohydrate diet
calories   1,960
   protein   70 gm.
   fat   63 gm.
   carbohydrate   277 gm.

2,000 calorie diabetic diet
calories   2,000
   protein   94 gm.
   fat   90 gm.
   carbohydrate   197 gm.

The first case emphasized the utility of drug therapy (Tolbutamide) in MS. Case number 2 is designed to illustrate the effects of *both* diet and drug treatment.

Case 2.—A 27-year-old man developed his first symptoms of multiple sclerosis only three years prior to admission. After several short remissions early in the course, his illness had progressed rapidly. On admission examination revealed a pronounced spastic quadriparesis, bilateral impairment of coordination, scanning speech, positive Babinski signs bilaterally, hypalgesia of the left lower extremity, and bilateral optic atrophy. [All of these are distinctly abnormal nerve function signs.] Results of laboratory examinations were within normal limits. An oral glucose tolerance test gave normal findings.

In the hospital three days after tolbutamide [0.5 Gm. per day] was started, the patient's strength began to improve. After several days he was able, for the first time in four months, to move his legs upward from the bed when lying in a supine position. The ataxia of the upper extremities also improved noticeably over an eight-day period. The patient was then given a high-carbohydrate diet [see table of diet composition] for five days. Within 48 hours after this diet was started he was worse in every respect. Slurring of speech, incoordination, and generalized fatigue were pronounced. He was then changed to a diabetic diet of 2,000 calories [see diet table] and, over a 16-day period, he developed increased strength in both upper and lower extremities. Coordination was also improved. Soon afterward the diet was again changed this time to a high carbohydrate type [see diet table]; the patient again started to weaken. After eight days on this diet he was so weak that he could not push his wheel chair and had increased difficulty with speech. At this point the tolbutamide dose was increased to 1.0 Gm. per day and the diet was changed back to a diabetic type consisting of 2,000 calories [see diet table]. Within 24 to 48 hours the patient began to improve dramatically. The generalized fatigue cleared, the spasticity of the lower extremities lessened, and there was increased objective strength in the upper extremities. He was able to transfer between wheel chair and bed more easily. The daily dosage of tolbutamide was then replaced with placebo capsules, and the high carbohydrate diet was again started. Over the next 23 days, the slurring of speech and spasticity of the lower extremities gradually increased in intensity. At this point, tolbutamide, 1.5 Gm. was given daily for 19 days. The strength of the upper extremities improved during this time.

Forty-eight hours after placebos were again substituted for the tolbutamide, the upper extremities developed considerable weakness and the speech grew fainter and more scanning. The patient was barely able to grasp objects, and it was extremely difficult to understand him.

Tolbutamide [0.5 Gm.] was then given daily for four days. Within two days the patient's grip was again strong, and his speech was noticeably improved. Placebo capsules were again substituted for the tolbutamide. After several days a right central facial paresis was noted for the first time, and it was evident that his speech was worse. [Parenthetic statements added].

There are common denominators in these two cases. Both have been clearly diagnosed as multiple sclerosis. The clinical symptoms and signs were improved and worsened by altering the carbohydrate metabolic picture. In simple terms, when these patients were viewed as diabetic and treated by diabetic techniques (drugs and/or diet) distinct improvement followed. Conversely, when these individuals were subjected to a diabetogenic (diabetes producing) diet, they got worse. This is particularly noteworthy since MS is usually not regarded as diabetes or in any way related to it.

Doctor E. M. Abrahamson (M.D.) has also observed a relationship between glucose tolerance and multiple sclerosis. In his observations of 126 cases of MS he was impressed by the fact that a functional hyperinsulinism existed in every person. This means that an excessive amount of insulin is released in the blood stream. According to Doctor Abrahamson, blood glucose levels below 70 mg. per cent within six hours after the consumption of 100 grams of glucose establishes the presence of hyperinsulinism. This chemical state is regarded as a pre-diabetic finding by many doctors. In other words, the person with low blood sugar today is more likely to be the high blood sugar (diabetic) of tomorrow!

A strict enforcement of a diet for hyperinsulinism was initiated for the following reasons: (1) it is high in fat, which depresses the oversensitive Islands of Langerhans, (2) the frequent feedings prevent drops in blood glucose after meals, (3) the carbohydrates are restricted to those that are slowly absorbed to avoid stimulation of insulin secretion by sudden increases in blood glucose, and (4) caffeine was also avoided for the same reasons as the simple carbohydrates. The Seale Harris Diet I was employed initially and was followed by Diet II after varying periods of time. These diets are so named in honor of the discoverer of this condition.

Although the therapeutic response to this diet has been variable, Doctor Abrahamson notes that the twelve treated cases show very little sign of multiple sclerosis.

SEALE HARRIS DIET I

On Arising.—Medium orange, half grapefruit, or juice [4 ounces].

Breakfast.—Fruit or juice [4 ounces]; 1 egg with or without 2 slices of ham or bacon; *only* 1 slice of bread or toast with plenty of butter; beverage.

2 Hours After Breakfast.—Juice [4 ounces] or fruit.

Lunch.—Meat, fish, cheese, or eggs, salad [large serving of tomato, lettuce, or Waldorf salad with mayonnaise or French dressing]; vegetables, if desired; *only* 1 slice of bread or toast with plenty of butter; dessert; beverage.

3 Hours After Lunch.—Glass of milk.

1 Hour Before Dinner.—Juice [4 ounces] or fruit.

Dinner.—Soup, if desired [not thickened with flour]; vegetables; liberal portion of meat, fish, or poultry; *only* 1 slice of bread if desired; dessert; beverage.

2 to 3 Hours After Dinner.—Glass of milk.

Every Two Hours Until Bedtime.—Juice [4 ounces], fruit, nuts [small handful], or ½ glass of milk.

Allowable Fruits.—Apples, apricots, bananas, berries, grapefruit, melons, oranges, peaches, pears, pineapple, tangerines. Fruits may be cooked or raw, with or without cream but *without sugar.* Canned fruits should be packed in water, unsweetened.

Allowable Vegetables.—Asparagus, avocado, beets, broccoli, Brussels sprouts, cabbage, cauliflower, carrots, celery, corn, turnips, cucumbers, egg plant, lima beans, onions, peas, radishes, sauerkraut, squash, string beans, tomatoes.

Allowable Juice.—Any *unsweetened* fruit or vegetable juice [4-ounce portions] except grape juice or prune juice.

Allowable Beverages.—Weak tea [teabag, not brewed]; Postum; Sanka.

Allowable Desserts.—Fruit; D-Zerta or other unsweetened gelatine; junket [made from tablets, not the mix].

Allowable Alcoholic and Soft Drinks.—Club soda, dry ginger ale, No-Cal beverages [except cola], whiskeys, and other distilled liquors.

Avoid Absolutely: Sugar, honey, candy, cake, pie, pastries, custards, puddings, ice cream; caffeine—ordinary coffee, strong brewed tea, "cola" beverages; potatoes, rice, grapes, raisins, plums, figs, dates, cherries; spaghetti, macaroni, noodles; wines, cordials, sweetened cocktails, beer.

[Milk, lettuce, mushrooms, and nuts may be taken as freely as desired. Use salt sparingly. Other condiments may be taken without restriction.]

SEALE HARRIS DIET II

Breakfast.—Fruit or juice [4 ounces]; cereal [dry or cooked] with milk or cream and/or 1 or 2 eggs with or without two slices of ham or bacon; *only* 1 slice of bread or toast with plenty of butter; beverage.

Lunch.—Meat, fish, cheese, or eggs; salad [large serving of lettuce, tomato, or Waldorf salad with mayonnaise or French dressing]; buttered vegetables, if desired; *only* 1 slice of bread or toast with plenty of butter; dessert; beverage.

Midafternoon.—Glass of milk.

Dinner.—Soup, if desired [not thickened with flour]; liberal portion of meat, fish, or poultry; vegetables; potatoes, rice, noodles, spaghetti, or macaroni [may be eaten in moderation *only with this meal*]; *only* 1 slice of bread, if desired; dessert or crackers and cheese; beverage.

Bedtime.—Snack [milk, crackers and cheese, sandwich, fruit, etc.].

All vegetables and fruits are permissible. Fruit may be cooked or raw, with or without cream but *without* sugar. Canned fruits should be packed *without* sugar.

Juice.—Any unsweetened fruit or vegetable juice, except grape juice or prune juice.

Beverages.—Weak tea [teabag, not brewed]; Postum; Sanka. May be sweetened with saccharine.

Desserts.—Fruit; D-Zerta or other unsweetened gelatine; junket [made from crushed tablets, not from junket mix].

Alcoholic and Soft Drinks.—Club soda, dry ginger ale, No-Cal beverages [except cola], whiskeys, and other distilled liquors.

Avoid Absolutely: Sugar, candy and other sweets, cake, pie, pastries, sweet custards, puddings, ice cream; caffeine—ordinary coffee, strong brewed tea, "cola" beverages; wines, cordials, cocktails, beer.

[Milk, lettuce, mushrooms, and nuts may be taken as freely as desired. Use salt sparingly.]

The successful treatment of multiple sclerosis has also been accomplished with a "low-fat diet." Since carbohydrate and fat metabolism are closely interrelated, metabolic improvement can be accomplished by manipulating either nutrient group.

Doctor Roy L. Swank (M.D., Department of Medicine, University of Oregon Medical School) describes his "low-fat diet" in the following fashion:

HOW TO GO AND STAY ON THE LOW-FAT DIET

Now that you have learned some of the history and reasoning behind the low-fat diet, you are ready to undertake the diet yourself.

The term, "low-fat diet," is precise and descriptive—the only item in your diet that will be restricted is the fat intake. You are limited to *35 grams or seven teaspoonsful* of fat per day, divided into *three teaspoonsful of animal or hard fat* or its substitutes and three teaspoonsful of fish *or vegetable oils* or their substitutes plus one teaspoonful of cod liver oil. This is both the maximum and minimum ration of fat for reasons of health and for palatability of the diet. If you are active and ambulant, *you should not eat less than the seven teaspoonsful daily.*

Following are lists of the fat and oil substitutes, which you will refer to often in the weeks ahead. [Special attention is called to the fact that margarine, shortening, and hydrogenated peanut butter are considered animal fat.]

Here are the substitutes for one teaspoonful of animal or hard fat:

- 2 ounces of beef sausage, veal, roast leg of lamb, ham, liver, chicken, or turkey
- 1 ounce of roast pork, pork chop, lamb chop, goose, duck bologna, salami, or liverwurst
- 3 slices of bacon, fried crisp and drained well
- 1 frankfurter
- 1 pork sausage
- 1 whole egg or 1 egg yolk [egg whites do not contain fat]
- 1 teaspoonful of margarine, shortening, or lard
- 2 teaspoonsful of hydrogenated peanut butter
- 1 small serving of canned pork and beans
- 2 level tablespoons of shredded coconut

Here are the substitutes for one teaspoonful of fish or vegetable oil:

- 1 teaspoonful of olive oil, corn oil, cottonseed oil, wheat germ oil, cod liver oil, or any other vegetable or fish oil which is liquid at room temperature
- 2 teaspoonsful of salad dressing or mayonnaise
- 2 teaspoonsful of non-hydrogenated peanut butter
- 2 ounces of salmon [fresh or canned], tuna fish, or trout
- 1 ounce of mackerel, herring, kippers, or sardines
- 4 small anchovies
- 5 olives
- 15 peanuts
- 7 almonds
- 2 walnuts
- 1 Brazil nut

The following foods are permitted in any quantity:
Boiled, broiled, or baked codfish, halibut, haddock, scallops, lobster, crab, and shrimp, as long as no fat or oil is used in the cooking process
Fresh or canned clams and oysters
All vegetables, including vegetarian baked beans
All fruits
All clear soups
All cream soups, if made with skim milk
Skim milk and buttermilk
Low-fat cottage cheese
All cereal products, including dry and hot breakfast cereals, white and brown bread and buns; spaghetti, macaroni, and other pastas [without sauce]
Jello and other gelatine desserts and salads
Desserts made from egg whites
Rice, tapioca, and cornstarch puddings made with skim milk and no egg yolk
Water ices
All fruit juices
All vegetable juices
Clear tea and coffee
Carbonated beverages
Jam, jelly, marmalade, preserves, and honey
Molasses
Maple syrup and corn syrup
Sugar
Seasonings

Foods permitted in limited quantities include soda, graham, and other crackers [not any containing cheese]; vanilla wafers; arrowroot biscuits; plain chocolate syrup [limited to one tablespoon daily; can be used for making chocolate frostings, chocolate cakes, milk shakes, plain chocolate sauce, hot chocolate, etc.]

Only two main categories of food are strictly forbidden—butterfat and chocolate [except the above-mentioned chocolate syrup.] The butterfat category includes whole milk, cream, butter, and cheese, and any foods containing these products, such as commercial pastries, pies, cakes, cookies, prepared cookie and cake mixes, doughnuts, ice cream, steamed puddings, cake puddings, and cream sauce. The chocolate category includes all candies containing chocolate, chocolate toppings and frostings, cocoa, hot chocolate, and other chocolate-flavored drinks, unless they are made with the allowed tablespoon of chocolate syrup. Avocados and eel also are considered to have too much oil to be included in this diet. It is best not to eat precooked frozen foods, such as French-fried potatoes, French-fried shrimp, and fish sticks, or canned spaghetti, with meat or meat sauce. Frozen foods have usually been precooked in shortening, and it is impossible to estimate the fat content of either these foods or canned spaghetti.

Each day you should consume all of the following:

[1] At least one egg. More eggs may be eaten if desired, but it should be remembered that each egg counts as one teaspoonful of animal fat. If you do not like eggs, as such, use them in cooking and baking, where you will not taste them but will receive nutritional benefit from them.

[2] Three glasses of skim milk or buttermilk.

[3] One multivitamin capsule.

[4] One teaspoonful of liquid cod liver oil. Probably no one likes the taste of cod liver oil and "burping" it is a universal experience. However, certain steps may be taken to minimize the unpleasantness. Keeping the oil cold in the refrigerator helps to kill the taste, or you may mix the oil with juice or wine to disguise the taste. Mint or orange-flavored cod liver oil is now on the market and some people find that this addition helps the palatability. Taking the oil just before retiring may lessen the "burping." Cod liver oil capsules should not be substituted, since the oil is taken not so much for its vitamin content [which you get from the multivitamin capsule] as for the essential fatty acids found only in the liquid form.

It is highly important that you include these four items just listed in your diet each day. They will help insure adequate daily amounts of protein, vitamins, and essential fatty acids which are necessary for energy and a feeling of well-being.

As an added insurance that you are receiving the proper amounts of proteins, you should use your animal or "hard" fat ration for eggs and meat. You should get your oil ration principally in the preparation of foods [all fats and oils used in this way must be counted as part of your daily ration] and in mayonnaise on sandwiches or in fish containing oil. It is important that fish or seafood be included in the daily menu, either in sandwiches for lunch or as snacks before dinner or between meals. This will assure you of a total protein intake of 75 to 90 grams daily, 45 grams of which will be animal in origin.

You may be surprised by some of the foods which are forbidden or limited on this diet. Most of us are aware that such foods as milk, cream, and butter contain fat, and we may be conscious of this fact as we eat them. But these "visible" fats actually make up only about 25 per cent of our normal daily fat intake. The other 75 per cent is made up of "invisible" fats—those added to our food in the cooking process, the shortening and eggs in cakes and pies, the milk in ice cream, and the fat contained in the lean parts of meat, to name only a few. For instance, cheese is usually considered a protein food, but it actually contains 50 per cent fat with a great amount of highly saturated fatty acids. *To make this diet effective you must become aware of the invisible fats as well as the visible ones and limit your fat intake accordingly.*

Virtually all foods contain some fat, but it would be impractical in day-to-day living to measure all of the small traces of fat which we consume. In the course of an ordinary day, you may eat as much as two teaspoonful of the unaccountable, immeasurable fats. For this reason, *it is particularly important that you weigh and measure the accountable fats listed above with accuracy and that you abstain completely from these foods on the forbidden list.*

How will you feel when you go on this diet? You may experience a certain amount of weakness and irritability during the first few months, but your body will quickly adjust and thereafter you will have as much or more energy than you had before. Occasional light snacks, such as a cup of tea and a few crackers, will help to banish the feeling of weakness during the adjustment period. If you work, carry some hard candy [*no* caramels], licorice, or crackers in your pocket or purse for a between-meal bite. You may crave these snacks anyway. Fats hold food in the stomach, and on the low-fat diet the stomach empties fairly rapidly. You will become hungry oftener than before, and a little food will help tide you over until the next meal. This hunger factor also helps you consume more carbohydrates, which is desirable if you wish to maintain your present weight. You may experience a slight weight loss at the beginning, but your weight will soon stabilize at a slightly reduced level, which in most cases is a desirable condition.

When Doctor Swank tabulated the clinical results of six and one-half years of low-fat dietary treatment, he found the following patterns. First, the early phase MS cases improved significantly. Second, the intermediate phase cases held their own. Third, the late phase cases slowly deteriorated. The overall performance of 121 cases of multiple sclerosis was tabulated in the following fashion:

PHASE OF MULTIPLE SCLEROSIS

	Early		Inter- mediate		Late		Totals	
Age of onset of multiple sclerosis [treated cases]	27.8		26.3		28.2		27.2	
Duration of multiple sclerosis before low-fat diet [years]	2.5		5.8		10.4		6.2	
Age when low-fat diet started	30.6		33.3		39.2		34.5	
Duration of low-fat diet [months]	76.0		87.8		78.0		80.0	
	No.	%	No.	%	No.	%	No.	%
Number of multiple sclerosis cases	56		25		40		121	
Improved	49	87.5	12	48.0	7	17.5	68	56.1
Unchanged	4	7.1	5	20.0	5	12.5	14	11.5
Deteriorated	3	5.3	8	32.0	28	70.0	39	32.2
Diet control:								
Good	42	75.0	13	52.0	25	62.5	80	66.1
Fair	14	25.0	12	48.0	15	37.5	41	33.9
Poor [excluded from analysis]	3		11		18		32	

Of the 56 cases with *early* MS shown in the table, 53 remained the same (7.1 per cent) or improved (87.5 per cent) during a period averaging nearly eight years. Such was the case for 17 (68 per cent) out of 25 with intermediate MS but only 12 (30 per cent) of 40 cases with *late* MS. Improvement was demonstrated in two ways. First, the frequency and severity of exacerbations (flare-ups of MS) were remarkably reduced. Second, the performance and neurologic status of patients was either improved or their deterioration was slowed for a period of observation on a low-fat diet lasting up to nine and one-half years.

In a final paper recently published in the Archives of Neurology, Doctor Swank assesses his experience in treating cases of multiple sclerosis with a low fat diet for more than 20 years:

> One hundred and forty-six patients with multiple sclerosis were placed on a low fat diet and followed an average of 17.1 years [14.5 to 19.7]. The course of disease in these patients was less rapidly progressive than in untreated cases available in the literature for comparison. There occurred a significant reduction in the death rate, in the frequency and severity of exacerbations, and in the rate at which patients became unable to walk and work. If treated early in the disease, before significant disability had developed, a high percentage of cases remained unchanged for up to 20 years. When treated later in disease, the disease usually continued to be slowly progressive. Patients who consumed the least amount of fat and the largest amounts of fluid oils deteriorated less than those who consumed more fat and less oil.

In this report Doctor Swank proposes that the fundamental cause of multiple sclerosis is an improper transportation of fat in the blood of patients who have inherited or acquired this defective transport mechanism. He notes that oils are moved primarily in the blood plasma (liquid part of the blood) but that fats such as butter fat, lard, and margarine are carried throughout the body attached to the red blood cells. This attraction may be responsible for the clumping or sludging of red blood cells after a fatty meal and may be fundamental to the development of multiple sclerosis.

Sludging of blood, a reduction in oxygen available to brain tissues, and an increased permeability (leaking) of the small blood vessels of the brain are possible steps in the genesis of the disease. The increased permeability or leaking would allow the toxic blood substances that emulsify fats to invade brain tissues and destroy the protective myelin sheaths of nerves (see What Is It?).

Improvement on the low-fat diet was significantly enhanced after 1951. It was at this time that animal and milk fats were severely restricted and a multiple vitamin capsule (Vitamins A, B complex, C, and D) was taken daily. Doctor Swank noted these alterations in the diet as follows:

The low-fat diet contained 30 to 40 grams of fat. Minor alterations, in the prescribed amounts and types of the lipid intake had taken place during the period of trial. During the first year of the study, from December 1948 to approximately December 1949, the diet contained 20 to 30 grams of fat, mostly milk and animal fat. During the next two years, the animal and milk fats were limited to 20 grams daily and to this were added 5 grams of cod liver oil and 10 to 15 grams of vegetable oil daily. In December 1951, milk fat was eliminated from the diet and the animal fat, including hydrogenated vegetable oils in shortening, margarine, and peanut butter was reduced to 15 grams a day. Fifteen grams of vegetable oil [corn oil, cottonseed oil, olive oil, soya bean oil, and safflower oil] and 5 grams of cod liver oil were retained in the diet. The protein intake was maintained at 50 to 90 grams daily, depending upon the weight, activity, and dietary habits of the patients. The balance of the caloric need was obtained from carbohydrates. In general, patients on this diet lost weight at first and stabilized their weights 5% to 10% under what is considered normal average weight. One multiple vitamin capsule containing Vitamins A, B complex, C, and D was taken daily, and the whole wheat bread was recommended. Skim milk or buttermilk was used by all patients as a protein supplement. Most patients ate at least one egg daily. The diet and many recipes substituting vegetable oils for animal and butterfats were furnished to the patient [Swank and Grimsgaard, 1959]. This detailed guide was followed by the patient.

The small amount of "invisible" fat contained in bread and many other foods were not accounted for in the diet. It was estimated that the average person consumed from 5 to 10 grams of fat from these sources daily. Therefore, the actual intake of animal or hard fat was probably 20 to 25 grams daily. It was felt that very little correction needs to be made for the oil intake. It was found easier to maintain a very low fat intake when the oil intake was allowed to vary freely according to desire and caloric requirements.

Doctor William F. Gerber, medical director of the Multiple Sclerosis Society of Colorado says that the Swank diet has been proved to be effective in the control of MS. The society has opened a clinic based on this dietary therapy in Denver.

On the surface, the suggestion of a "low-fat diet" appears to be quite different from the "low-carbohydrate" recommendations of Doctor Sawyer and Doctor Abrahamson. Actually, the two regimes are quite similar if a few facts are clarified.

National levels of consumption of fat and simple carbohydrates (sugar and syrups) have been noted to be strikingly similar ($r=0.81$) for 41 countries. This is, in part, because many foods high in sugar are also high in fat content (doughnuts, cake, pie, ice cream, cookies, puddings, candies and other sweet pastries). Therefore, the reduction in fat consumption and the elimination of butterfat and chocolate by Doctor Swank's "low-fat diet" produces a significant lowering of the refined carbohydrate (simple sugar, syrup and pastries) content of the diet. These simple carbohydrates are the foods primarily restricted by Doctors Sawyer and Abrahamson.

SUMMARY

There is hope for the person with multiple sclerosis! Diet, as a therapeutic tool, certainly should be included on the basis of this evidence.

The dietary regimes referred to in this chapter propose a restriction of saturated fats and the simple carbohydrates (sugar and syrup). In the light of the dietary evidence just shown and the definition outlined on page 18, simple sugars and saturated fats should be viewed as susceptibility factors in multiple sclerosis. It may be recalled from Chapter Three that the primary alteration in the average American's food intake during the past 80-100 years has been a marked reduction in starch and a dramatic (more than double) increase in the consumption of simple sugars (primarily sucrose or table sugar) and syrups.

It must be admitted that these studies are incomplete. Much more knowledge is needed about the cause and cure of MS. In the meantime, what should the patient with multiple sclerosis do? It seems reasonable that the procedures outlined here should be tried for three reasons. First, the dietary regimes outlined here are harmless. Secondly, the MS patient has no other choice since the disease is admittedly incurable. Finally, these dietary regimes at least offer some hope for these incurables!

The most sensible approach for the MS patient is to consult a physician knowledgeable in these techniques.

REFERENCES

1. Abrahamson, E. M. *An investigation of the role of hyperinsulinism in multiple sclerosis; preliminary report.* New York State Journal of Medicine 54: #11, 1603-1608, June 1, 1954.
2. Alter, M. *Clinical evaluation of possible etiologic factors in multiple sclerosis.* Neurology 18: #2, 109-116, February 1968.
3. Alter, M. *Etiologic considerations based on the epidemiology of multiple sclerosis.* American Journal of Epidemiology 88: #3, 318-332, November 1968.
4. Alvarez, W. C. *Multiple [disseminated] sclerosis.* The Register and Tribune Syndicate, Inc., 1968.
5. Harrison, T. R., Adams, R. D., Bennett, T. L., Jr., Resnik, W. H., Thorn, G. W., and Wintrobe, M. M. *Principles of internal medicine.* Fifth edition. 1966. New York, McGraw-Hill Book Company.
6. *Multiple sclerosis in the United States.* Statistical Bulletin Metropolitan Life Insurance Company 48: #6, 6-10, June 1967.

7. Sawyer, G. E. *Treatment of multiple sclerosis with tolbutamide; a preliminary report.* The Journal of the American Medical Association 174: #5, 470-473, October 1, 1960.
8. Swank, R. L. *A biochemical basis of multiple sclerosis.* 1961. Springfield, Illinois, Charles C. Thomas.
9. Swank, R. L. and Grimsgaard, A. *Low-fat diet; reasons, rules, and recipes.* 1959. Eugene, Oregon, University of Oregon Books.
10. Swank, R. L. *Multiple sclerosis—twenty years on low-fat diet.* Archives of Neurology. 23: #11, 460-474, November 1970.
11. Yudkin, J. *Dietary fat and dietary sugar in relation to ischemic heart disease and diabetes.* Lancet 2: #7349, 45, July 4, 1964.

5

Is There Hope
For the Alcoholic?

INTRODUCTION

THE ANSWERS TO these five questions are very important to the alcoholic and his or her family!

What is it?
What causes it?
How common is it?
What cures it?
Is there more hope?

WHAT IS IT?

Alcoholics are people with a disease that can be defined in medical terms. Alcoholics are addicted to alcohol and are unable spontaneously to quit drinking. Though they can endure without a drink for varying periods of time, they inevitably return to their drinking habits. The greater the need to cease drinking, the more difficult it is to stop. Thus, the alcoholic has lost the power of choice in drinking. His will power with regard to alcohol is practically nonexistent. Even the most powerful desire to stop drinking is generally of no avail.

There is a common characteristic to all alcoholics: they cannot start drinking without developing the phenomenon of craving. The first drink causes something to happen physically and mentally which makes it virtually impossible to stop. The idea that somehow and some day they will control and enjoy drinking is a great obsession of many problem drinkers. The persistance of this illusion is astonishing, and many pursue it to insanity and death.

According to the World Health Organization (WHO), "alcoholics are those excessive drinkers whose dependence on alcohol has attained such a degree that they show a noticeable mental disturbance or an interference with their mental and bodily health, their interpersonal relations, and their smooth social and economic functioning; or who show the prodromal signs of such developments."

The American Medical Association (AMA) as well as the World Health Organization and many other professional groups have come to regard alcoholism as a specific, complex disease or illness. The AMA definition is as follows:

> Alcoholism is an illness characterized by preoccupation with alcohol and loss of control over its consumption such as to lead usually to intoxication if drinking is begun; by chronicity; by progression; and by tendency toward relapse. It is typically associated with physical disability and impaired emotional, occupational, and/or social adjustments as a direct consequence of persistent and excessive use.

In short, the American Medical Association regards this illness as a type of *drug dependence* of pathologic extent and pattern, which ordinarily interferes seriously with the patient's total health and his adaptation to his environment.

Authorities have described three stages of alcoholism: (1) excessive drinking, (2) alcohol addiction, and (3) chronic alcoholism. Although the many signs and symptoms of these phases may not represent the course of a particular alcoholic, it is a realistic picture of progression for most of these unfortunate people.

PHASES IN ALCOHOLISM

STAGE OF EXCESSIVE DRINKING

1. More time spent in social drinking
2. Drinks more nights of the week
3. Sneaks drinks
4. Takes stronger drinks than companions
5. Adopts strategies to get more drinks
6. Preoccupied with drinking
7. Drinks to get relief from tension
8. Increased tolerance
9. Guilt over drinking
10. Social failures excused to himself and to others with fabricated explanations
11. Needs drink to perform adequately at work or socially
12. Feels drink has become a necessity
13. Increased guilt feelings

STAGE OF ALCOHOL ADDICTION

1. Onset of alcoholic amnesias [memory losses]
2. Greater frequency of amnesias
3. Loss of control—compulsive drinking
4. Reduction in interests
5. Drop in work efficiency
6. Absenteeism
7. Drunk in the daytime
8. Reproof from employer or relatives
9. Low self-esteem
10. Remorse
11. Compensatory bragging and generosity
12. Financial extravagance
13. Deceives family, debts made
14. Increasing social isolation
15. Aggressive outbursts
16. Wife takes over more responsibilities
17. Deterioration in relation with wife
18. Paranoid misinterpretations
19. Self-pity
20. Justifies drinking with self-deceptions
21. Reduction of sexual drive

22. Morbid jealousy
23. Drunk at weekends
24. Loss of job .
25. Breakup of family
26. Morning tremulousness
27. Morning drinking
28. Conceals supplies of liquor
29. Repeated attempts to stop drinking
30. Suicidal impulses and attempts
31. Neglect of meals

STAGE OF CHRONIC ALCOHOLISM

1. Physical and mental symptoms dominate
2. Loss of appetite, poor food intake
3. Continuous drinking
4. Tolerance diminishes
5. Prolonged confused thinking
6. Use of cheap wines and methylated spirits
7. Delirium tremens
8. Goes to AA or seeks medical treatment
9. Serious physical diseases

One of the most frustrating characteristics of alcoholism is the inability of the drinker (at any stage of his illness) to accept or recognize that he is in serious trouble despite overwhelming evidence that this is the case. To help the drinker admit that he has problems with his drinking (the first step in any recovery program) Dr. Robert V. Seliger of Johns Hopkins University Hospital has developed a series of twenty questions related to drinking. The individual is reminded that only he can determine whether or not he is an alcoholic. It has been the experience of the membership of Alcoholics Anonymous if he answers "yes" to as few as three questions, he can be reasonably certain that alcohol has become, or is becoming, a problem for him. Although this approach has all the inherent weaknesses of any self-appraisal procedure, it has nevertheless proven to be a most useful and widely accepted diagnostic tool.

The twenty questions are as follows:

1. Have you lost time from work due to drinking?
2. Has drinking made your home life unhappy?
3. Do you drink because you are shy with people?
4. Has drinking affected your reputation?
5. Have you gotten into financial difficulties because of your drinking?
6. Do you turn to lower companions and an inferior environment when drinking?
7. Does your drinking make you careless of your family's welfare?
8. Has your drinking decreased your ambition?
9. Do you want a drink "the morning after"?
10. Does your drinking cause you to have difficulty sleeping?
11. Has your efficiency decreased since drinking?
12. Has drinking ever jeopardized your job or business?
13. Do you drink to escape from worries or troubles?
14. Do you drink alone?
15. Have you ever had a complete loss of memory as a result of drinking?
16. Has your physician ever treated you for drinking?
17. Do you drink to build up self-confidence?
18. Have you ever been in an institution or hospital on account of drinking?
19. Have you ever felt remorse after drinking?
20. Do you crave a drink at a definite time daily?

Some A.A. groups have added other questions to this list of twenty. One publication (*A.A., A way of life,* Division of Alcoholism, 715 State Office Building, Montgomery, Alabama 36104) has expanded the number to forty. For diagnostic purposes, however, the twenty questions are adequate to indicate or predict a drinking problem.

WHAT CAUSES IT?

Confusion has always surrounded the etiology of alcoholism. It has been the subject of endless speculation and considerable earnest investigation. Most authorities now agree that there is no single cause but rather a complicated interplay of psychologic, sociologic, and physiologic factors (American Medical Association).

Psychologic Factors: Psychopathologic factors are regarded as being of great importance in the initiation and development of alcoholism. However, they fail to answer many questions concerning etiology and progression. For instance, few persons, if any, survive childhood without emotional trauma, often of a severe type; and many endure early emotional disturbances or deprivations without crippling signs of immaturity. Depression may persist throughout life, yet without alcoholism.

Any emotional disorder seen in an alcoholic may be observed in patients with other illnesses who make adequate adjustments. Psychoanalytic resolution of basic conflicts by no means cures the alcoholic, and conditioning treatments aimed at helping him unlearn his patterns have not been especially successful. To ignore these factors, however, would be to court defeat in any treatment program.

Sociologic Factors: Alcohol serves vastly different functions within societies, cultures, subcultures, ethnic, and religious groups. Attitudes concerning its use range from permissiveness to total abstinence. The purposes for which alcohol is used include religious, culinary, psychic, ceremonial, hedonistic, traditional, social and medicinal. Standards of acceptability applied to the manner or pattern of drinking vary according to occasion, sex, cultural background, social class, and the particular circumstances. Thus, sociologic factors have an influence upon the use of alcohol and are important in the etiology and development of alcoholism, as well as in its treatment.

No single sociologic factor has been identified that has a uniquely causative effect. However, the influence of sociologic forces is broad, and cannot be excluded from consideration in any successful therapeutic effort.

Physiologic Factors: Until quite recently, the role of physiologic factors in alcoholism has received limited interest from scientific investigators.

But refinements in research and controlled experimental investigations are providing greater insight into this aspect of alcoholism. Many hypotheses have been advanced concerning the physiologic status of the body and alcoholism. These include the following:

1. Allergy to alcohol, the grain from which an alcoholic beverage is made or other ingredients or contaminants.
2. Abnormal sugar metabolism, especially a reactive or functional hypoglycemia [low blood sugar] or hyperinsulinism [high insulin blood level].
3. Hormone deficiency of the thyroid, pituitary, or adrenal glands or the gonads.
4. Dietary or metabolic deficiency of vitamins, minerals, enzymes or other nutrients.
5. Liver dysfunction.
6. Sensitivity to a basic foodstuff which is relieved by alcohol.
7. Defective function of an "alcohol appestat" in the hypothalamus, causing uncontrollable thirst for ethanol.
8. Imbalance of acetycholine and receptor sites in the ascending reticular formation of the brainstem, leading to need for alcohol to bind with an excess of receptor sites.

Thus, physiologic factors cited as causative agents in alcoholism have been related to allergy, abnormal carbohydrate metabolism, hormone imbalance, nutrient (vitamin, mineral, enzyme) deficiency, liver dysfunction, and functional or metabolic disorder in the brain.

According to Shadel Hospital and Enzomedic Laboratories, Inc., of Seattle, Washington, the biologic basis of excessive or progressive drinking involves a deficiency of the enzyme, DPN (diphosphopyridine nucleotide). It is also known as nicotinamide adenine dinucleotide (NAD), which is a co-enzyme obtained by extraction from yeast.

The biologic relationship of this enzyme to the initiation and development of alcoholism is explained in these terms:

> It is of paramount importance to realize that people differ in their resistance to systemic poisons, the sting of a bee, or in their reactions to the poison of ivy, even in their ability to digest such a common food as sugar.
>
> Our research indicates that alcohol is a drug that is addictive in varying degrees for approximately 20 per cent of the population in the United States, but functions as a nonaddictive tranquilizer for the remaining 80 per cent under ordinary, voluntary circumstances. Alcohol consumed by the average person passes through his body, and does not leave an addictive "hook." However, some people are not able to remove the toxic by-products from their system.
>
> The toxic [poisonous] residue causes a disturbance in the body including tension, anxiety, irritability and thirst. These effects are temporarily alleviated by more of the sedative, alcohol, so such people continue to drink relentlessly
>
> The need for additional sedative, alcohol, is intensified if the person also attacks his nervous system with nicotine.
>
> The alcohol enters the body as a sedative, but if it is not metabolized properly, it becomes an irritant, "fire water." To the drinker this cycle is often initially imperceptible, increasing gradually in intensity over the years. This sequence is caused by an enzyme dysfunction found most frequently in North America among the American Indians and those of Irish, Scandinavian, French, English and German descent, in that order. This enzyme dysfunction is genetically transmitted and precludes drinking alcohol moderately.
>
> *Of course, the genetic deficiency may not be transmitted to all descendants.*
>
> Famines, diet, climate, which shape a people's genes over centuries, have been mentioned as possible causes for this enzyme dysfunction.

A diet high in carbohydrates and low in vitamins, minerals, and protein may create a predilection for drinking alcohol —at least in rats, according to investigators from the Loma Linda (California) University School of Public Health.

In animal studies, the chemical imbalance created by such a diet seems to lead to a craving for ethanol. Working with 96 rats who had the choice of drinking water or a 10 per cent ethanol solution in water, 30 rats became moderate drinkers in five weeks on the high carbohydrate diet.

The 30 rats were divided into three groups for another 16-week study. One remained on the high carbohydrate diet; another received the same diet with vitamin and mineral supplements; and the third group ate a balanced human diet.

The rats on the high carbohydrate diet consumed an average of 49.5 ml. of ethanol per week (the equivalent of more than a quart of 100 proof whiskey a day for an adult man). Rats who ate the high carbohydrate diet with vitamin-mineral supplements drank an average of 16.8 ml. of ethanol per week, and those on the balanced human diet consumed a weekly average of 7.0 ml. of ethanol.

One-fifth of the rats did not develop any taste for alcohol during the initial five-week study (96 rats) on the high carbohydrate diet. The addition of sugar to the ethanol solution, however, turned these rats into the heaviest drinkers of all. They consumed up to 70 ml. of ethanol per week each when continued on the high carbohydrate diet for the final 16 weeks of the study. When half of these rats were given a balanced diet, they began at once to consume much less alcohol.

HOW COMMON IS IT?

Alcoholism ranks with cancer and heart disease as one of the nation's three leading killers, according to Marion J. Wettrick, a member of the Board of Directors of the North American Association of Alcoholism Programs.

The annual prevalence of alcoholism in the United States has been estimated to be between 4.1 and 5.2 per cent, 20 years of age and older. This would tend to support the estimate that one in twenty adults (5 per cent) is afflicted with problem drinking.

With approximately 120 million adults in the 20 and above age bracket, an alcoholism incidence of 5 per cent would yield approximately 6,000,000 alcoholics. Various estimates of the number of alcoholics in the United States range from four to seven million. It is quite possible that these figures are conservative. In fact, Morris E. Chafetz of the American Psychiatric Association claimed in a recent U.S. Senate testimony that the nation's alcoholics number nine million. Many are convinced that the incidence is rising, for the consumption of alcohol is increasing.

Whatever the actual incidence and prevalence of alcoholism, no one can doubt the magnitude of the medical, social, and economic consequences to society. Seen in terms of the tragedy, unhappiness, misery, suffering, and waste of life, even the most calloused observer must be concerned.

The approximately 6,000,000 alcoholics in this country adversely affect the lives of 25,000,000 people! Not only does the alcoholic hurt his family (psychologically, sociologically and many times, physically), he is frequently involved with total strangers. For instance, figures from the National Safety Council point to alcohol as a causative factor in about one-third of the automobile accidents fatal to adult pedestrians. According to figures published by the Schick Safety Razor Company and Associated Employers Insurance Company, the economic losses to this country from alcoholism are staggering:

> "If the 6,000,000 addicts stopped consuming an average of $2.90 daily or $7.2 billion worth of alcohol annually and increased their earnings by $5,000 yearly, the total additional purchasing power would amount to $34.5 billion."

Alcoholism is also a burden to all law enforcement agencies. The Federal Bureau of Investigation reports indicate that more than 40 per cent of all arrests are for drunkenness, the greater proportion of which presumably involve alcoholics.

WHAT CURES IT?

Although alcoholics are treatable patients, their recovery rate in relation to the total number of alcoholics is very low. This is, in part, related to its many causes. Although much therapeutic emphasis has been placed upon the psychologic and sociologic factors, relatively little interest has been shown toward correction of the physiologic flaws (see *What Causes It?*). Also, it is quite difficult for an alcoholic to admit alcoholism, to desire abstinence, and to accept help toward this end. In most instances the alcoholic cannot reach this decision.

Alcoholics Anonymous has been more successful in helping alcoholics than any other organization or therapeutic approach. However, their promise of recovery through the famous "TWELVE STEP" program is only to those who are willing to take STEP NUMBER ONE—"We admitted we were powerless over alcohol—that our lives had become unmanageable." Unfortunately, very few alcoholics take this STEP. Most local AA groups are listed in the telephone directory. Al-Anon and Al-Ateen groups have also been formed to help the spouses and children of the alcoholic.

IS THERE MORE HOPE?

There is much more hope for this nation's four to seven million alcoholics if the diagnosis and treatment of physiologic flaws or defects are pursued. Where diet and nutritional emphasis have been given in the treatment of alcoholism, recovery is only a little short of fantastic!

Without citing the vast number of research and clinical

efforts which confirm nutritional inadequacy in the alcoholic, the following defects are exhibited (these and other physiologic flaws were noted in a previous section—*What Causes It?*):

1. Multiple deficiencies involving most of the essential vitamins, minerals, and amino acids.
2. Abnormal sugar metabolism, especially a reactive or functional hypoglycemia [low blood sugar]. This results, in part, from too much insulin which is secreted following a rapid rise in the circulating blood glucose [sugar] level. The rapid rise occurs following the consumption of table sugar and foods or drinks high in sugar or starch. Evidence provided by six-hour glucose tolerance tests in alcoholics shows that hypoglycemia exists in from 70 to 90 per cent.
3. Deficiency of the enzyme DPN [diphosphopyridine nucleotide], also known as nicotinamide adenine dinucleotide [NAD].

The multiple deficiencies of vitamins and minerals created by subsistence on alcohol are readily reversed following the administration of therapeutic quantities of the essential vitamin-mineral nutrients in a tablet or capsule form. Such therapeutic multivitamin-mineral supplements should be taken with breakfast, lunch, and dinner (or supper). These do not require a prescription and can be obtained from any drug store, health food store, or pharmacy. For this purpose, the greater number of vitamins and minerals which can be combined in a single pill, tablet, or capsule, the better!

The provision of general nutritional support can be accomplished with a diet high in complete (animal) protein, moderate to high in total fat (roughly balanced between saturated and unsaturated fats), and very low in simple or readily assimilated carbohydrates (sugar, high starch foods). Such a diet also prevents the broad swings in blood glucose (both high and low levels) which are found in many alcoholics and which seriously impair their physical and emotional stability. Many versions of this diet have been published under a variety of names or terms. All are modifications of the "Seale Harris Diet" (see this diet in Chapter Four, Multiple Sclerosis). Both the "Hypoglycemia Diet" and "Anti-Hypoglycemia Diet" are good examples of diets designed to correct the low blood sugar syndrome.

HYPOGLYCEMIA DIET

[Harry M. Salzer, M.D., 6056 Montgomery Road, Cincinnati, Ohio 45213]

Immediately On Arising: 4 to 6 oz. orange juice, frozen or fresh; or one medium orange. [Orange juice or orange allowed *only* once a day on arising.]

Breakfast: Fruit or 4 oz. juice; 1 or 2 eggs with or without two slices of bacon or ham; only one slice of any bread or toast but with plenty of butter or oleomargarine; beverage.

2 Hours After Breakfast: 8 oz. juice or milk.

Lunch: Meat, fish, cheese or eggs, salad [large serving lettuce, tomato, or Waldorf Salad with mayonnaise or French dressing]; vegetables if desired; only once slice of any bread with butter or oleomargarine; dessert; beverage.

2 or 3 Hours After Lunch: 8 oz. milk.

1 Hour Before Dinner: 4 oz. juice.

Dinner: Soup if desired [not thickened with flour]; *liberal* portion of meat, fish, or poultry; vegetables; only one slice of bread if desired but with plenty of butter or oleomargarine; salad; dessert; beverage.

Every 2 Hours Until Retiring: 8 oz. milk and/or a small handful nuts or 1 or 2 saltines but must be with cheese or dietetic peanut butter.

If Wakeful During Night: Eat a high protein snack.

Meat, or milk, or nuts, or 4 oz. of allowable juice may be taken hourly through the day if underweight or if symptoms are severe.

HYPOGLYCEMIA DIET
[*Food and Drink Allowed*]

Allowable Vegetables: Fresh, frozen or canned: artichoke, asparagus, avocado, beets, black-eyed peas, broccoli, Brussels sprouts, cabbage, cauliflower, carrots, celery, corn, cucumbers, eggplant, garlic, kale, lentils, lettuce, lima beans, mushrooms, okra, onions, peas, peppers, pumpkin, radishes, sauerkraut, soy beans, spinach, squash, string beans, sunflower seeds, tomatoes, turnips, water cress. [Corn, lima beans, lentils and peas are least desirable].

Allowable Fruits: Fresh or cooked or unsweetened frozen or canned: Apples, apricots, berries, cherries, fresh coconut, grapefruit, kumquats, lemons, limes, mango, melon, papayas, peaches, pears, pineapple, and tangerines—with or without cream but *without sugar.* Sweeten with saccharin, Sucaryl or Sweeta.

Allowable Juice: The following if unsweetened: Apple, grapefruit, [orange juice or orange only on arising], pineapple, tomato, vegetable, Vegemato, V-8. Sweeten only with saccharin, Sucaryl or Sweeta. Knox gelatin may be added for protein.

Allowable Beverages: Above juices, dietetic carbonated drinks except cola, creamed or plain buttermilk, Kaffir tea [obtainable at health food stores], milk, vichy, Fizzies, Fresca.

Allowable Desserts: Fruit, unsweetened gelatin, Dezerta fruit flavors, junket from tablets only, and the following dietetic products: candy [except chocolate], gum, fruits, ice cream, jelly or puddings—sweetened with saccharin, Sucaryl or Sweeta but not sugar, syrup or honey. Dietetic maple syrup permitted.

HYPOGLYCEMIA DIET
[*Absolutely None of the Following*]

Sugar, Honey, Candy Including Chocolate, Other Sweets Such As: cake, chewing gum, Jello, pastries, pie, puddings, sweet custard, sweet jelly or marmalade, and ice cream.

Caffeine: Ordinary coffee, coffee substitutes [Sanka and Decaf], tea, beverages containing caffeine [Coca Cola, Pepsi Cola, other cola drinks], Ovaltine, Postum, hot chocolate.

Drinks and Juices: No ordinary carbonated drinks. No grape, prune or other juices than those listed above.

Fruit: Bananas, dates, dried fruits, figs, grapes, persimmons, plums, prunes, raisins.

Starches: Macaroni, navy and kidney beans, noodles, potatoes, rice, spaghetti and ravioli.

Alcoholic Beverages: Beer, cocktails, cordials, wines.

Medications Containing Caffeine Such As: Anacin, A.P.C., A.S.A.

COMPOUND, B.C., Caffergot, Coricidin, Empirin Compound, Fiorinal, Four Way Cold Tablets, Salfayne, Stanback, Trigesic. [Plain Aspirin or Bufferin permitted].

Read the label on every can of juice, fruit, vegetable, meat and other products. Select only those containing no syrup, honey or sugar. These can be found at the dietetic counters in all large markets.

Do not change timing, type, or amount of food.

ANTI-HYPOGLYCEMIA DIET
[Hypoglycemia Foundation, Inc., Scarsdale, New York 10583]

Foods Allowed: All meats, fish, shell fish and fowl. Dairy products [eggs, milk, butter and cheese. Also recommended—1 large glass of acidophilus milk daily].

Salted nuts [excellent between meals.]

Peanut butter [if no sugar has been added].

Sanka, weak tea, and sugar-free sodas.

Soybeans and soybean products.

Low carbohydrate bread in moderation [2 slices daily], preferably made chiefly of combined oat, soya, gluten, and Jerusalem artichoke flours.

All vegetables and fruits not listed below.

Olives, pickles, mushrooms, salads, vinegar, mayonnaise.

Artificially sweetened and "non-sugar" foods prepared commercially for the diabetic or "weight-watcher" [including ice cream].

Unstrained orange juice [preferably whole segments] is useful as a source of Vitamin C and potassium. Even when used in moderation, orange juice may contain too much sugar for some patients; in this case other sources of these essential elements must be used.

Potato chips may be used tentatively if they are thin, heavily salted and saturated with fat, in moderation of course.

Foods to Avoid: All sugars and honey. Potatoes, corn, macaroni, spaghetti, rice, peas, lima beans, baked beans.

Regular bread, pie, cake, pastries, candies.

Dates and raisins and other dried fruits.

Cola and other sweet soft drinks.

Coffee and strong tea.

All hot and cold cereals [except occasionally oatmeal].

All alcoholic beverages [narcotics, and drugs which act as stimulant or depressant, are to be avoided].

The importance of proper diet cannot be overemphasized. The diet essentially consists of strict elimination of *rapidly absorbed carbohydrates* in order to obviate the sudden rise in blood sugar with its subsequent fall.

A hearty breakfast and between-meal and bedtime feedings of milk, salted nuts, cheese, meat or fruit are advised to prevent any slackening off of blood sugar levels, which is prone to occur two to three hours after eating. Generous use of salt is encouraged because of the tendency to "salt waste" which results in sodium depletion. During hot weather salt tablets should be used to replace the loss caused by perspiration.

In an estimate of the impact of nutritional attack (therapeutic multivitamin-mineral supplements and the hypoglycemia-type diet) on alcoholism, Doctor Roger J. Williams (Professor of Bio-chemistry, University of Texas) reported that at least 50 per cent would dramatically benefit and that all others would receive some help. Doctor Williams said:

I know of scores of individuals who have made at least partial trials with tremendous success. In some cases every testimony is that abolishment of appetite [for alcohol] has been complete and lasting, something little short of miraculous. In other cases, the help has been less dramatic. I know of no one who has attempted seriously to follow a sensible nutritional regimen who has not appeared to receive substantial benefit. . . . Because of the success I have witnessed in the nutritional combat against alcoholism, I have not the slightest hesitation in recommending to alcoholics and to those who may have the beginnings of an alcohol problem, that they try the nutritional approach.

Doctor Allen A. Parry, Chief of Alcoholic Service, The Morristown Memorial Hospital, Morristown, New Jersey, claims that with the combined approach of medication, counselling, and nutrition, good results are obtained in fifty to seventy per cent of the total number of alcoholics seen. He emphasizes that the element in this approach so frequently slighted by other agencies is the nutritional factor. Doctor Parry cautions that with nutritional support it is much easier for the alcoholic to stay sober, even though their disease is not cured but only controlled. In other words, they are still alcoholics.

The treatment of alcoholism as an enzyme deficiency with nicotinamide adenine dinucleotide (NAD) has also produced dramatic results. The records of 14,000 patients treated for alcohol addiction at Shadel Hospital, Seattle, Washington, since 1940 indicate that 66 per cent remain totally abstinent after the initial treatment.

The most exciting nutritional innovation in treating alcoholism is the "megavitamin" approach. In an initial report, Doctor Russell F. Smith (M.D., Consultant, Brighton Hospital, Detroit; Guest House, Lake Orion, Michigan; Michigan State Social Services and Boy's Training School) noted dramatic recovery following massive niacin (Vitamin B_3) therapy. In a midpoint progress report on massive vitamin therapy of 507 alcoholics in Michigan for 1967-1968-1969, Doctor Smith continues to be enthusiastic. This report to Bill W., a co-founder of Alcoholics Anonymous, stated:

January 1970

Dear Bill W.:

I'm glad to act upon your request that I update my preliminary 1967 Report on "Massive Niacin Therapy of Alcoholics in Michigan," covering 507 alcoholics for periods of six to twenty months.

All these patients had previously been longtime treatment failures with histories including multiple in-patient therapy, state mental hospital therapy, private psychotherapy, legal punitive therapy, counseling, and Alcoholics Anonymous. As documented in this earlier report, the results were even then very promising.

We now have *two additional years* of careful follow-up on this group. Hence, the three-and-one-half-year results here described are accurately and fully documented.

Of our original cases, only 70 have been lost by attrition.

Most of the dropouts represented B-3 treatment failures. This leaves us now (1970) with 437 cases who have been under observation on niacin therapy for three years or more. In terms of sobriety, these 437 alcoholics can be seen in the following categories:

Sober (3 years plus)	138
Sober (2 years plus)	256
Improved (fewer relapses, etc.)	43
TOTAL	437
Failures and deaths	70
TOTAL (original group)	507

Stating these results in percentages: Of the original group, 78 percent have been continuously sober from two to three years or more; 8 percent are improved, and only 14 percent have left the group.

In their first year of treatment, (1966) all of the original group was placed *exclusively* on massive niacin. It is therefore noteworthy that 138 of our 507 original patients have since continued on massive niacin alone, meanwhile maintaining practically perfect sobriety. All of this group are sober three years or more—as of January 1, 1970.

At the close of our first year, however, approximately 256 of the group were still experiencing emotional difficulties and some relapses. In these situations, niacin dosage was greatly increased and supportive medication was found to be helpful. These people are now sober for two years or more, and the need for supportive medication has greatly lessened or disappeared.

This leaves only forty-three who continue to have relapses into drinking or experience severe emotional difficulties. Most of them have improved, but their progress has been very slow. They do have fewer relapses, and their tensions are diminished. In addition to very large amounts of niacin they continue to use considerable medication.

Of the few deaths that have occurred, only three were due to cardiac failures. Considering that the original group was 80 percent male and most of them in an age bracket of high coronary incidence, this was astonishing. It appears to be a very strong confirmation of Boyle's report on niacin and the heart in your 1968 publication.

Meanwhile, we have observed no adverse liver damage among our group that could be traced to the use of massive niacin.

However, we have discontinued niacin in a few instances of uncontrollable diabetes or persistent intestinal problems.

Certainly this record points up the value of continuous megadoses of niacin. In my view, little if anything could have been achieved with this very difficult group of patients had the B-3 Therapy not been used. Most certainly this has been crucial to their recovery.

Nevertheless, we should not conclude that niacin alone is a wholesale remedy for alcoholism. The fact is, that niacin has made other treatment effective; treatments as various as supportive medicine, personal counseling, psychiatry, and Alcoholics Anonymous. In fact, the majority of our group now maintain their sobriety in AA.

Hospitalization, plus B-3 Therapy, plus counseling, plus AA, are adding up to unprecedented results among alcoholics who otherwise would have had a very bad prognosis. Taken together, these resources constitute a new treatment model of great promise.

At this point it may be beneficial to present a more detailed statistical tabulation of what has happened. Here is our classified table:

	Poor	*Fair*	*Good*	*Excellent*	*Total*
Outpatient Group (1967)	18	70	109	42	239
Outpatient Group (1968)	3	45	123	62	233
Outpatient Group (1969)	0	20	125	69	214
Hospital Group (1967)	40	19	111	46	216
Hospital Group (1968)	21	45	87	57	191
Hospital Group (1969)	0	20	91	63	174
Sanitarium Group (1967)	8	9	20	15	52
Sanitarium Group (1968)	3	8	23	19	50
Sanitarium Group (1969)	0	3	25	21	49

Our criteria for evaluation have been as follows:

POOR RESPONSE

1. No objective or subjective change.
2. Continued unaltered drinking pattern.
3. No change in sleep pattern.
4. No change in mood or affect.
5. No change in supportive medication needs.
6. Psychological state compatible with Menninger Scale—Classes One and Two.

FAIR RESPONSE

1. Reduced rate of recidivism.
2. Improved sleep pattern.
3. Decreased supportive medication needs.
4. Psychological state comparable with Menninger Scale—Class Three.

GOOD RESPONSE

1. Marked reduction in recidivism.
2. Normal sleep pattern.
3. Marked reduction in supportive medication needs.
4. Absence of extreme depression or euphoria.
5. Absence of emotional "dry drunks."
6. Psychological state compatible with Menninger Scale—Class Four.

EXCELLENT RESPONSE

1. Total abstinence from alcohol intake for two or more years.
2. Mood stability.
3. No need for supportive medication other than Vitamin B-3.
4. Psychological state compatible with Menninger Scale—Class Five.

Every patient has been evaluated in the fall of each year. A serum cholesterol and serum lipid was obtained whenever possible. In most cases our subjects were examined personally. This was usually done by the professional personnel originally responsible for their treatment. Where this desirable procedure was not possible, our evaluation was carried out by mail, and then augmented by third party evaluation, if obtainable.

Our considerable experience now makes possible several pertinent observations:

(A) All members of the study-group sample have normal serum lipid values and, most surprisingly, normal cholesterol. As previously observed, there were only three deaths due to cardio-vascular causes. (B) Niacin therapy has a significant effect in reducing alcohol tolerance. (C) Niacin therapy has demonstrated a significant effect on sleep patterns. (D) It has also demonstrated very significant mood-stabilizing effects, and has all but eliminated the recurrent flashback emotional "dry drunk," in a group where such phenomena could be expected in high frequency.

Comparison of yearly tabulations suggest that when niacin is effective, this effectiveness can improve with prolonged use. Where however the effect is minimal, motivation to take the vitamin drops, and the patient himself discontinues the medication.

Our future plans are as follows:

1. To continue the present study of our 507-member group for two more years—making five years in all.

2. We now have access to 3673 other patients in various stages of niacin-nicotinic acid therapy, in addition to our original 507 cases. When sufficient time has elapsed we shall make a full report on this much larger sampling.

3. We also plan a formal cross-over, double-blind study to be carried out in the two sanitarium groups available to us. This study will be completed by 1972.

4. We have also begun basic investigation into five-OH Tryptophan metabolism in the brain stem, since nicotinic acid itself is a byproduct of serotonin and norepinephrine production. Multiple research reports suggest these two neurohormones play a major role in mood and in sleep. Quite possibly these same neurohormones may be implicated in the mechanisms of alcohol tolerance and withdrawal.

At present the clinical observations resulting from our study have suggested basic research which could lead to vastly increased knowledge of the mechanisms of alcohol tolerance and withdrawal, and very well of the disease of alcoholism.

Sincerely,
Russell F. Smith, M.D.

P.S. At the beginning of our study, some of the group was started on nicotinamide instead of niacin. However, this was discontinued because the effects of very large doses of niacin were far superior.

For those who flush severely on niacin, we recommend 4 mg. periactin daily. Since the flushing due to histamine release is no different for one or 200 mg. than for one gram, we find it best to start patients on 4 grams of niacin daily.

Doses in our present study group are now stabilized and range from 4 to 20 grams, according to need with an average dosage of 6 grams in four divided doses after meals and at bedtime. One gram of ascorbic acid in two divided doses are given to offset increased consumption of niacin.

Although, clinically, niacin produces a remarkable physical and mental improvement (and/or stabilization) in most alcoholics, its chemical action is poorly understood. However, the mechanism of niacin in checking hypoglycemia may offer a clue. It was previously noted that six-hour glucose tolerance tests reveal a relative or functional hypoglycemia in seventy to ninety per cent of alcoholics tested. This depression of blood glucose levels by excessive quantities of insulin and/or weak adrenal glands which cannot immediately elevate the blood level to normal produces a variety of signs and symptoms—vertigo, headaches, fatigue, exhaustion, drowsiness, muscular pains, leg cramps, insomnia, nightmares, irritability, nervousness, nervous breakdown, lack of concentration, constant worry and anxiety, depression, forgetfulness, phobias, suicidal thoughts, weakness, lightheadedness, fainting, tremors, cold sweats, inside trembling, incoordination, staggering, convulsions, tachycardia (fast heart rate), palpitation (pounding heart beat), blurred vision, allergies, itching or crawling sensations, neurodermatitis, arthritic pains, gouty arthritis, gastrointestinal symptoms, loss of libido.

The psychologic and physiologic experience of hypoglycemia is quite different for different people. In addition to many combinations of the above signs and symptoms, alcoholics experience a craving for alcohol and the so-called "dry drunk."

Confirmation of the megavitamin approach in the treatment of alcoholism also comes from The North Nassau Mental Health Center (1961 Northern Boulevard, Manhasset, Long Island, New York 11030). Doctor David R. Hawkins, who directs a staff of eighteen psychiatrists, two psychologists, two psychiatric social workers, seven secretaries and five volunteers, reports that most of the 300 alcoholics treated since 1966 are now good parents, and effective citizens. In addition to vitamin megadosage (niacin, 4 grams or more per day; ascorbic acid, 4 grams per day; pyridoxine, 50 mgs. per day; vitamin E, 800 international units per day) four times each day, a diet was employed to correct functional hypo-glycemia (hyperinsulinism) or so-called low blood sugar.

In a letter to the authors of this book, Doctor Hawkins describes his successful clinical approach in these words:

> The last two years has seen a very rapid expansion of our work and the incorporation of many new ideas and concepts. Our approach has continued to grow in the direction of searching for certain biochemical abnormalities in patients and correcting these first before we go further with any psychological approaches to clinical problems. We have also discovered that in a very sizable percentage of patients the biochemical abnormalities are of paramount importance and once they are corrected recovery takes place almost spontaneously. Many more disorders than alcoholism appear to us to be physical as well as mental and spiritual. The great majority of our patients we have found have biochemical and metabolic problems which have been extremely important in preventing their recovery from their illness.
>
> The human mind does not exist in a vacuum but operates as a molecular function of the brain. Alterations of the molecular concentration of the substances normally present in the human body can greatly alter mental functioning. This important concept was presented by twice Nobel prize winner Professor Linus Pauling in April, 1968 in an article entitled "Orthomolecular Psychiatry."
>
> To many of us now working in this field Pauling's concept very accurately describes what we were doing and is now being generally adopted. We are editing the first book on Orthomolecular Psychiatry which will be published in 1970 entitled ORTHO-MOLECULAR PSYCHIATRY: Treatment of Schizophrenia, which will include contributions by twenty-three different authors and will include a chapter on Schizophrenics Anonymous, which was the first sizable patient group to utilize this new approach in helping to solve their problems. Schizophrenics Anonymous emphasizes the physical, mental and spiritual aspects of that illness. It comes as no surprise to AA's that most and perhaps all the serious mental illness are physical, mental and spiritual and the patients are unlikely to recover unless all three approaches are combined. This is, however, a new concept in psychiatry. We can see now that psycho-analysis was not wrong, it merely wasn't enough to cure the more serious illnesses such as alcoholism or schizophrenia or any of the other serious addictions.
>
> Many psychoanalysts intuitively knew this to be so and Existentialism was added which included a recognition of man's spiritual

needs, especially in the here and now. This helped many people come to grips with their condition, live with it and function but still the patient did not feel cured. Psychopharmacology contributed a great deal. It eliminated symptoms, made conditions much more bearable and the tranquilizers and anti-depressants did much to alleviate suffering and enabled some people to recover, or compensate for still undetected impairments. Recognition of the importance of detecting these biochemical impairments and correcting them and giving the patients total recovery has been the main contribution of Orthomolecular Psychiatry and we can expect many further advancements in this field in the future.

Since 1966 we have now treated over 2,000 patients utilizing this overall approach of whom approximately 300 were alcoholics. In the alcoholic, three problems appeared over and over again and were either responsible for the patient's failure to recover or were responsible for slips or prevented full recovery despite having obtained sobriety. The first problem we check for is the use of any of the hypnotics, barbiturates or the so-called minor tranquilizers. Although very few of the patients were actually addicted to these substances the effect of taking even minute amounts, even quite infrequently, seriously interfered with the patient's sobriety and brought about subtle alterations in thinking and feeling if not outright slips. The most common offenders were Librium, Miltown, Valium, Doriden, Noludar, Placidyl and Quaalude. In every single case where these were used the effect was noticeably deleterious.

Functional hypoglycemia (hyper-insulinism) or so-called low blood sugar, was another factor commonly present and previously undetected, which accounted for many failures to recover. These patients immediately felt better as soon as they were taken off sugar and sweets, which we found to be more conclusive then obtaining a five-hour glucose tolerance test in the laboratory. Many of the alcoholics who did get the five-hour glucose tolerance test reported that during the course of the test they began to develop symptoms which they recognized they had had for many years and which usually preceded drinking. Quite a few patients who have been sober for considerable lengths of time have reported periodic depressions, feelings of tension and anxiety and recurrent desires to drink and correction of the hypoglycemia completely eliminated these symptoms in the great majority.

The third large problem we discovered in alcoholics to play a very important part in delaying or preventing recovery were the presence of multiple perceptual distortions as revealed by administering the HOD Test. The HOD Test is a test for alterations of perceptions such as touch, taste, hearing, vision and perception of bodily parts with associated feelings. There are also alterations of the perception of time and space which may be altered and which also show up on the HOD Test. Most recently drinking alcoholics will show a High HOD score initially but this rapidly returns to normal following cessation of drinking. In many of the patients that we saw who had been unable to get sober or who were sober but miserable, an elevated HOD score persisted. The alterations in perception are thought to be due to alterations in brain function on a chemical basis due, perhaps, to abnormalities of adrenaline metabolism as described by Drs. Hoffer and Osmond and many others. In some patients the HOD score was so high as to give the patient symptoms of schizophrenia so that it was hard to say whether the patient had schizophrenia complicated by alcoholism or alcoholism which had developed into schizophrenia. Although hallucinations are common during the DT's, many of these patients were continuing to have hallucinations long after they had stopped drinking.

The great majority of these patients also had functional hypoglycemia as well and their overall condition was quite severe. These patients responded very well to a combination of Vitamin B-3 in doses of four grams or more per day plus ascorbic acid in doses of four grams per day with the addition of 50 mgs. a day of pyridoxine and in many cases Vitamin E, 200 international unit capsules, four times a day. The theory behind the megavitamin approach is that the megavitamins correct the abnormal breakdown of the adrenaline into toxic byproducts which are the cause of the perceptual alterations and the elevated HOD score. In any case correcting hypoglycemia, taking patients off harmful drugs and placing them on megavitamins sometimes with the addition of one of the phenothiazines drugs brought about remarkable recovery.

These perceptual problems appear to occur very often in the young alcoholic especially, so that we now screen every alcoholic patient with the HOD test. Many patients who are on niacin reported a greatly diminished desire to drink as well as alleviation of other symptoms.

Within the last year we have a new chapter of Schizophrenics Anonymous on Long Island and we now have a chapter of American Schizophrenia Foundation and many of the AA's who have rather marked perceptual distortions identify with both SA and AA. In fact, many of the SA groups which have recently formed around the country have been started by the AA's who had perceptual problems. The growth and development and success of the SA groups was reported in World Medical News in a special article on Schizophrenics Anonymous in December, 1969. Quite a few alcoholics have entered AA through SA which helped them correct their perceptual problems to the point where they were able to recognize and deal with their alcoholism and do something positive about it.

The SA groups have all located doctors in their community with whom they work who are either knowledgeable about this approach or interested in learning to work with it. This would also be best for the AA's who want to add this approach to their own recoveries. The number of doctors now utilizing this approach is proliferating at such a rate that finding suitable medical assistance should not be difficult.

The American Schizophrenia Foundation of 610 South Forest Avenue, Suite 6, Ann Arbor, Michigan 48104, has an expanding referral list of doctors using the megavitamin approach.

SUMMARY

Try these questions. Remember, there is no disgrace in admitting that you have a health problem. If you do have a problem, the important thing is to do something about it.

1. Have you ever tried to stop drinking for a week [or longer] only to fall short of your goal?
2. Do you resent the advice of others who try to get you to stop drinking?
3. Have you ever tried to control your drinking by switching from one alcoholic beverage to another?
4. Have you taken a morning drink during the past year?
5. Do you envy people who can drink without getting into trouble?
6. Has your drinking problem become progressively more serious during the past year?
7. Has your drinking created problems at home?
8. At social affairs where drinking is limited, do you try to obtain extra drinks?
9. Despite evidence to the contrary, have you continued to assert that you can stop drinking on your own whenever you wish?

10. During the past year have you missed time from work as a result of drinking?
11. Have you ever blacked out during your drinking?
12. Have you ever felt you could do more with your life if you did not drink?

Alcoholics Anonymous World Services, Incorporated, asks, what's your score? Did you answer YES four or more times? If so, chances are you have or will have a serious drinking problem. *If you want help, Alcoholics Anonymous is for you.* They are as near as your telephone and will be glad to show you how they were able to stop drinking.

There is also a remarkable new hope for the alcoholic. Nutritional therapy has been demonstrated to be beneficial at any stage of alcoholism. In fact, the physical and emotional improvement which occurs will bring many alcoholics into such groups as Alcoholics Anonymous that would or could not have made this move without nutritional assistance.

The restriction of dietary carbohydrate, an increase in protein and unsaturated fat and the utilization of megadoses of niacin and ascorbic acid provide the physical and mental stabilization in many alcoholics which is so desperately needed at the beginning of sobriety.

From the evidence presented, it appears that sugar and other highly processed carbohydrates are detrimental to the alcoholic and that vitamins, minerals and protein are beneficial. Hence, based on the earlier definitions (Chapter Three), these carbohydrates must be viewed as susceptibility factors in alcoholism. Conversely, protein, vitamins and minerals may be regarded as resistance agents.

Although the consumption of megadoses of Vitamin B_3 is quite safe, there are several contraindications and annoying side effects. These are effectively summarized in a useful booklet on Megavitamin Therapy by the Better Health Center, 5629 State Road, Cleveland, Ohio 44134:

CONTRAINDICATIONS

Though the megavitamin therapy can be used in combination with any other drugs and treatments, there are some cases where the physician has to choose one compound instead of the other, raise the dosages slowly, or watch for certain changes. These are:

Peptic ulcer or hyper-acidity patients should observe the diet and medication prescribed by their physicians, and if they cannot tolerate niacin, should use it with antacids, or they can use other preparations, like buffered niacin, or niacinamide.

High blood pressure patients who use reserpine type medications may experience nausea and considerable drop in blood pressure when using high dosages of niacin. This might not be dangerous but could be very inconvenient.

Liver function test might show false indications, if someone is on niacin. Therefore, niacin should be discontinued for a week before this or other sensitive tests (like glucose tolerance test) are taken. (Smoking, too, disturbs glucose tolerance tests.)

SIDE EFFECTS

Vitamin B-3: Niacin, but not niacinamide, causes flush at the beginning.

Your skin turns pink as if you had a sunburn. You might feel your skin tighten and you may have some prickling feeling or itching. This flush might start almost immediately, or hours after you take the pill, and at the beginning it might last for a few hours. Some people like it; others, especially children, cannot tolerate it. If you drink a glass of cold milk after taking the tablets, it reduces the flush. Or take niacin with the solid part of your meal. Regulate your schedule so that there is little flushing in public. Your physician can prescribe 4 mg. periactin but take this only when you wish to eliminate flush or other side effects. Even if you get accustomed to niacin and do not flush any more, it starts again if you neglect taking niacin for a few days and then take it again. If you cannot get accustomed to it, change to niacinamide that does not cause flush. Neither flush nor the other side effects are dangerous but might be very inconvenient to some people.

About five people out of 100 get headaches. This can be remedied by ordinary painkillers.

A few people develop nausea and rarely even vomiting. This can be remedied by periactin or by using buffered niacin or niacinamide. Or doctors can prescribe another form of Vitamin B-3, as Complamin (available in the U.S. from Riker Corporation, in

Canada from Elliot-Marion). Antacids can be used to relieve acidity. . . .

If skin rash develops, it can be cured by 4 mg. periactin or 50 mg. benadryl, taken when needed with niacin.

If shock-like reaction occurs with a drop of blood pressure, it can be easily controlled by posture: taking the first dose while lying on a bed.

Allergic reactions might occur, due not to niacin, but to the filler [starch, etc.] used to make the tablets. In this case, products of another company should be tried out, because they might use a different kind of filler that does not cause allergy.

Many times the inconvenient side effect can be stopped by changing from niacin to niacinamide or vice versa.

REFERENCES

1. Adrenal Metabolic Research Society. *Hypoadrenocortism, the endocrinologic approach to the etiology and treatment of functional hypoglycemia as a factor in adrenocortical dysfunction—medical management of hypoglycemia states including allergy, alcoholism and emotional disturbance.* Hypoglycemia Foundation, Inc., Scarsdale, New York 10583.
2. Adrenal Metabolic Research Society of the Hypoglycemia Foundation, Inc., P.O. Box 26, Scarsdale, New York 10583. *Hypoglycemia and me?*
3. *Alcohol—who is allergic? Schick Safety Razor Company,* Culver City, California; Enzomedic Laboratories, Inc., 126 S. W. 157th Street, Seattle, Washington 98166.
4. Alcoholics Anonymous World Services, Inc. *Is A.A. for you?* 1954. P.O. Box 459, Grand Central Post Office, New York, New York 10017.
5. *Alcoholism: a growing medical-social problem.* Statistical Bulletin, Metropolitan Life Insurance Company 48: #4, 7-10, April 1967.
6. American Medical Association. *Manual on alcoholism.* 1967.
7. *Authorities on alcoholism urge new national program.* The Alabama Baptist 135: #23, June 4, 1970.
8. Cahalan, D. and Cisin, I. H. *American drinking practices: summary of findings from a national probability sample. I. Extent of drinking by population subgroups.* Quarterly Journal of Studies on Alcohol 29: #1, 130-151, March 1968.

9. Department of Public Health and Mendocino State Hospital, Talmage, California.
10. Kessel, N. and Walton, H. *Alcoholism*. 1965. Penguin Books, Inc., Baltimore, Maryland.
11. Lipscomb, W. R. *Survey measurements of the prevalence of alcoholism as seen by the practicing physician, a review of five studies*. Division of Alcoholism, State of California.
12. Medical News. *High carbohydrate diet affects rat's alcohol intake.* Journal of the American Medical Association 212: #6, 976, May 11, 1970.
13. Rouse, K. A. *Detour; alcoholism ahead.* Kemper Insurance, 4750 Sheridan Road, Chicago, Illinois 60640.
14. Salzer, H. M. *Hypoglycemia diet.* 6056 Montgomery Road, Cincinnati, Ohio 45213.
15. The Christopher D. Smithers Foundation [New York, New York] and the Clayton Foundation Biochemical Institute [The University of Texas, Austin]. *A symposium on the biochemical and nutritional aspects of alcoholism.* October 2, 1964.
16. *The vitamin B-3 therapy: a second communication to A.A.'s physicians from Bill W.*, P. O. Box 451, Bedford Hills, New York 10507.
17. U.S. Department of Health, Education and Welfare, Office of Program Analysis. *Health, education and welfare trends,* 1965 edition. Part One, p. 12.

6

Is There Hope for the Glaucoma Patient?

INTRODUCTION

FOR THOSE WITH glaucoma, the answers to these five questions are important!

What is it?
What causes it?
How common is it?
What cures it?
Is there more hope?

WHAT IS IT?

Glaucoma, in its more common form, can destroy vision slowly and painlessly, sometimes without giving any warning signs or symptoms to its victim until most of the sight is gone. Although there are many types of glaucoma, one feature is common to all—increased pressure within the eyeball.

A healthy eye has an optimal or favorable pressure within it called the intraocular (within the eye) pressure. Without this force, the eye would collapse like a leaking balloon. Intraocular pressure varies somewhat in different persons and even from day to day in the same eye. This variation is similar to that of the blood pressure in that a fairly wide range is considered acceptable.

When the pressure increases to such a degree that damage to structures within the eye occurs, the condition is called *glaucoma* or hypertension of the eye (also commonly termed hardening of the eyeball). There is no direct relationship, however, between high blood pressure (arterial hypertension) and glaucoma (hypertension of the eye).

Although it is possible to become overly glaucoma-conscious, there are certain signs and symptoms which should induce one to be examined by an ophthalmologist (an eye doctor). Early detection is important because vision lost as a result of glaucoma is never regained (except to a very minor degree). It is a question of keeping what vision a patient has rather than any hope for appreciable improvement. While glaucoma can sneak up without warning, the following symptoms or danger signals can occur—*rainbow-colored rings (halos) around lights, a narrowing of the visual field, frequent changes in eyeglass prescriptions without visual improvement, abnormally poor vision in dim light, fuzzy or blurred vision which may come and go, vague headaches or eye aches, particularly after watching movies or television in darkened rooms, watering or discharge of the eye, any change in eye color, clouding of the cornea and hardness of the eyeball.* Another warning is a family history of glaucoma. Relatives of those with glaucoma have five or six times as much of this eye ailment as persons without glaucoma in the family.

WHAT CAUSES IT?

The front portion of the eye between the lens and the cornea holds a clear watery fluid called the aqueous humor. Throughout a person's life, this watery substance is constantly produced within this tiny chamber, flows through it to nourish the cornea, and then drains through a minute natural canal.

For reasons not yet completely understood by science, this drainage canal may become blocked.

If this happens, the aqueous humor backs up and pressure within the eyeball builds up. This force is transmitted to the retina (on the back side of the eye). The retina contains sensitive nerve cells and fibers that relay light stimuli through the optic nerve to the brain. Increased intraocular pressure can cause destruction of these cells; and, with each cell destroyed, a portion of the field of vision is lost forever. Eventually all sight may be gone.

Glaucoma usually begins with the loss of peripheral or side vision, then slowly closes in until only straight-ahead vision is left, then none at all. A person may be unaware of the loss of side (lateral, peripheral) vision because he can see straight ahead with 20/20 central vision. It is generally concluded that an elevated pressure over a long period of time is necessary to produce visual field defects. While this may be correct for many patients who develop such loss of sight, it should be noted that there are also individuals with elevated pressure for long periods of time who do not develop visual field loss. Since so little is actually known concerning the cause of glaucoma, host resistance and susceptibility factors in the latter group might provide some clues (see Chapter Two). In fact, malnourishment of the disc (where the optic nerve attaches to the eyeball) because of impaired blood circulation has been suggested.

Basically, there are two divisions of glaucoma, *primary* and *secondary*. Although much is known about what happens in primary glaucoma, the fundamental cause or causes remain a mystery. Primary glaucoma occurs in both eyes and is called "primary" for the simple reason that it is apparently not "secondary" (or due) to some other disorder. The conditions which result in secondary glaucoma are almost too numerous to list. As the term implies, the high pressure within the eye is a result of some disease, tumor, inflammation, or injury. Secondary glaucoma is frequently limited to one eye.

Within the *primary* division there are three types of glaucoma. *Chronic* glaucoma is the most common and is the type usually referred to in this chapter. It is the classic sneak thief of vision and is an extremely deceptive disorder. *Acute* glaucoma is uncommon and attacks suddenly and painfully. The pressure must be reduced immediately or blindness will result. Although it presents a critical emergency, cure is more often achieved (medically and surgically) than with the other types. Finally, *infantile* glaucoma is a rare congenital type requiring surgery.

HOW COMMON IS IT?

Numerous detection surveys have shown that the incidence of glaucoma (mostly undetected) is about 2 per cent of the people over 40. This percentage increases progressively with age. It is estimated that approximately 2,000,000 American adults already have glaucoma and that half of them are not aware of it. The incidence and prevalence of glaucoma in blacks is almost twice as high as in white persons. In those with a positive family history of this affliction, screening surveys have shown that almost one of every ten adults examined had glaucoma. This observation suggests a possible genetic influence. However, the mere fact that something runs in families does not preclude its being environmentally inspired.

Although glaucoma is primarily a disease of those over forty years of age, disturbances in sugar metabolism encourage its development much sooner. Generally, the duration of diabetes mellitus is directly related to the intraocular tension.

In other words, the longer the duration, the higher the introocular pressure. Thus, juvenile diabetes can produce abnormally high tensions in the first two decades of life.

Next to cataracts, glaucoma is the leading cause of blindness. There are about 54,000 men and women in this country who are blind in both eyes and an additional 185,000 blind in one eye from this disease. According to health authorities, the blind population has been increasing at nearly twice the rate of the general public. Not only is this trend continuing, but it is believed that the increase will accelerate.

WHAT CURES IT?

Any mention of the treatment of glaucoma must be, for the most part, quite general, for no two cases are exactly alike. The therapy by one ophthalmologist may vary somewhat from that of another. Yet both may achieve similar results. However, it is of great importance that glaucoma treatment usually be looked upon as a control and not a cure! In other words, *glaucoma is controlled rather than cured!*

In acute (rather severe but of short duration) glaucoma, drug relief is usually followed by surgery. For chronic glaucoma (not severe and of a long duration), restoration of vision already lost due to nerve degeneration cannot occur. Thus, therapy is designed to preserve the remaining sight. Astute patient control is necessary in chronic glaucoma since treatment is lifelong and the disease is slowly progressive. Initially, miotic drugs (eye-drops) effectively increase the outflow of aqueous humor to keep the intraocular pressure down. Other eye-drop drugs may also be used to reduce the formation of this fluid and thus aid in suppressing the pressure. Failure to control the pressure with these agents may be followed with an oral drug designed to decrease the rate of aqueous humor formation. At some point in the progression of chronic glaucoma, a decision is usually made to improve the aqueous outflow by a surgical procedure. Where surgery does not control the intraocular pressure, progression to blindness is almost inevitable.

As additional aids in the control of glaucoma, the following instructions are applicable to most patients:

1. Follow the advice of your ophthalmologist to the letter. This is by far the most important thing to keep in mind. Return for checkups when advised.

2. Notify your ophthalmologist immediately if you should develop pain or redness of the eye or sudden blurring of vision. If intense itching accompanies swelling and redness of the eyelids and eyes, tell your ophthalmologist promptly. It may mean that you have developed an allergy to a medicine that you are using.

3. Avoid excessive use of stimulants such as coffee and tea. It is preferable that you give up all such stimulants. If you drink coffee, however, one-half to one cup a day should be your limit. You may have caffeine-free coffee.

4. Avoid excessive amounts of fluid intake at any one time. In hot weather, excessive perspiration may necessitate your drinking larger amounts of fluids than usual. Do not drink three or four glasses at any one time, however; spread them out.

5. Avoid excessive smoking. It is not known with certainty how much damage smoking causes in cases of glaucoma; but there is enough evidence to indicate that smoking does cause some harm.

6. You should attempt to lead as tranquil a life as possible. Avoid emotional upheavals so far as possible.

7. Avoid prolonged periods of darkness, such as several hours a week at motion pictures. Do not use sunglasses too much. In the very bright sun, however, shaded glasses do no harm.

8. Most ophthalmologists feel that the ordinary use of the eye does no harm insofar as glaucoma is concerned. This means that you may read, sew, and watch television without fear of damage to your eyes.

9. When you consult your family physician or your surgeon, tell him that you have glaucoma. He will avoid giving you certain drugs that might adversely affect your glaucoma.

10. If you move or have any other reason to change your care to another ophthalmologist, request that your old record be sent to him.

11. Carry an identification card at all times. It is advisable to carry

this card with information as to your condition, just as a patient with diabetes does. There are several reasons for this. If one is found unconscious from an accident or for some other reason, the examining physician, on seeing the card, will realize that the person's small pupils are due to the use of drops in the eyes. Unless this information is known, the small pupils may be misinterpreted. On seeing the identification card, the physician will be on guard, too, about administering drugs that might adversely affect the glaucoma. Your ophthalmologist can secure these cards from the National Foundation for Eye Care.

REMEMBER THAT THE MOST IMPORTANT FACTOR IN THE TREATMENT OF YOUR GLAUCOMA IS TO FOLLOW YOUR OPHTHALMOLOGIST'S ADVICE TO THE LETTER.

IS THERE MORE HOPE?

At a recent meeting of the Roman Ophthalmological Society in Rome, Italy, four Italian physicians gave evidence of an exciting breakthrough in glaucoma treatment. Doctor Michele Virno and coworkers cited human evidence that the intraocular pressure in glaucomatous eyes could be dramatically reduced by an oral dose of Vitamin C (ascorbic acid)! This report was immediately published in the United States by the Eye, Ear, Nose and Throat Monthly.

The initial approach by these investigators was to evaluate the effect of a single oral dose of Vitamin C (0.5 grams of ascorbic acid per kilogram, 2.2 pounds, of body weight) upon the intraocular pressure in patients with different kinds of glaucoma. For example, a person weighing 150 pounds would receive 35 grams of Vitamin C. This megadose is over 500-fold the amount generally held to be an optimal daily intake. Doctor Virno and his associates observed a highly significant drop in pressure for all patients. This table is a summary of their findings (eye pressure is expressed in millimeters of mercury):

Type of glaucoma	No. of eyes	Average maximum eye pressure reduction [expressed in millimeters of mercury]
Chronic simple glaucoma		
initial pressure 50-69	7	25.0
initial pressure 32-49	7	19.0
initial pressure 20-31	11	6.5
Acute glaucoma		
partial angle closure	3	28.5
complete angle closure	4	10.5
Hemorrhagic glaucoma	2	17.0
Secondary glaucoma	5	11.5

It was noted that the intraocular pressure reached its lowest point about four to five hours after taking the single dose of Vitamin C. This low point was maintained for more than eight hours. It was also observed that the blood Vitamin C level, which was very low in the beginning, reached its highest point as the pressure reached its lowest level. This blood level was about eight to ten times greater than initially. After five hours, the blood Vitamin C level began to decrease.

Since most patients treated with the single load of Vitamin C developed disorders of the stomach and diarrhea, Doctor Virno decided to divide the single dose into several smaller ones. Thus, amounts of 0.10 to 0.15 grams per kilogram (2.2 pounds) of body weight were given three to five times a day. Thus, the 150 pound person mentioned earlier would be given about seven grams five times each day. Although this produced mild stomach discomfort and diarrhea at the beginning, these symptoms disappeared after three to four days.

With these smaller doses, which were administered daily for periods up to forty-five days, it was possible to obtain acceptable intraocular pressure in many patients. This happened in some individuals whose pressure could not be controlled with oral drugs (such as Diamox) or eye drops (miotics such as 2 per cent pilocarpine).

Doctor Virno and his team expressed hope that others will use Vitamin C in the treatment of glaucoma. Although the mechanisms are not completely understood, the administration of ascorbic acid in the smaller doses three to five times a day is very effective and perfectly safe!

SUMMARY

Professor G. B. Bietti, Director of the Eye Clinic of the University of Rome, where this research has been conducted, recently offered these conclusions concerning the Vitamin C treatment:

1. Vitamin C at high dosage is a very effective hypotonic agent for intraocular pressure, not only when administered by intravenous injection [sodium ascorbate: from 0.4 to 1 gramme per kilogram of body weight], but also when given by mouth [ascorbic acid: 0.12 to 0.5 gramme per kilogram of body weight].
2. The hypotonic effect on the eye of ascorbic acid by mouth lasts longer than other agents which have an osmotic action when given by both oral and intravenous routes [including sodium ascorbate] although the action of ascorbate lasts longer than that of urea, mannitol and glycerol given by mouth.
3. Ascorbic acid given by mouth has various intensities of action depending on the individual patients and the types of glaucoma and seems more effective in cases of chronic open-angle glaucoma.
4. Ascorbic acid has proven equally active whether given in a single dose of 0.5 gramme per kilogram of body weight or in fractional doses during the day.
5. It has also been proved that the hypotonic action of ascorbic acid on the eye can be prolonged practically indefinitely, at least for the period observed in patients so treated [seven months] by the daily administration of divided doses of 125 mg. per kilogram of body weight two, three or four times a day. Normal intra-ocular tension could be obtained by treat-

ment with ascorbic acid by itself, or in association with topical antiglaucomatous medication [miotics], on occasions when miotics by themselves were unable to control the tension. . . .

In some cases the lowering of the intra-ocular tension caused by prolonged treatment with ascorbic acid persisted for several weeks after the treatment had been stopped. Sodium ascorbate given by intravenous injection acts predominantly by osmotic dehydration of the eyeball, although it is possible that there is a different additional action of the ascorbate itself or of the ascorbic acid liberated from it in the body.

The other possible mechanism of action of ascorbic acid on intra-ocular tension, as proven by tonographic investigations and those with a suction cup [modified by Bucci], seems to be a chemical one causing a diminished production of aqueous by the ciliary epithelium.

An additional hypotonic mechanism, acting very possibly through a decreased production of aqueous, could be the shift of blood pH towards the acid side. . . .

The medical profession emphasizes that the medical and surgical treatment of glaucoma should be looked upon as a control and not a cure. In many people, however, the control is not adequate to prevent the disease from progressing. Since the oral administration of Vitamin C has been reported to be highly effective in reducing high intraocular pressures to a normal or near normal level, there are many good reasons for trying it:

1. Vitamin C is nontoxic [safe] in the dosage recommended for glaucoma.
2. Vitamin C is a cheap and convenient way to treat glaucoma.
3. Vitamin C, taken orally, does not produce the degeneration of eye and body tissues that occurs with the strong eyedrops and oral medications used in treating glaucoma.
4. The preservation of sight may be accomplished with Vitamin C even after all drugs and surgery have failed.

Based on the earlier definitions (Chapter Two, page 16) and the evidence presented here, Vitamin C must be regarded as a resistance agent in glaucoma.

The sensible course for the patient with glaucoma is to consult an eye doctor regarding the possible use of this treatment.

REFERENCES

1. Becker, B. and Shaffer, R. N. *Diagnosis and therapy of the glaucomas.* Second Edition. 1965. St. Louis, C. V. Mosby Company.
2. Bietta, G. B. *Further observations on the value of osmotic substances as means to reduce intra-ocular pressure.* Transactions of the Ophthalmological Society of Australia 26: 61-71, 1967.
3. Chandler, P. A. and Grant, W. M. *Lectures on glaucoma.* 1965. Philadelphia, Lea and Febiger.
4. Frydman, J. E., Clower, J. W., Fulghum, J. E., and Hester, M. W. *Glaucoma detection in Florida.* The Journal of the American Medical Association 198: #12, 1237-1240, December 19, 1966.
5. Georgia Society for the Prevention of Blindness. *Early detection can control glaucoma.* Journal of the Medical Association of Georgia 57: #10, 481, October 1968.
6. Information Office, National Institute of Neurological Diseases and Blindness, NIH. *Cataract and glaucoma; hope through research.* Public Health Service Publication #793, Health Information Series #99, 1968.
7. Knopf, M. M. *Glaucoma therapy simplified.* Journal of the Mississippi Medical Association 10: #9, 457-461, September 1969.
8. Levene, R. Z. *Glaucoma; annual review.* Archives of Ophthalmology 81: #3, 421-440, March 1969.
9. Levene, R. Z. *Glaucoma; annual review.* Archives of Ophthalmology 83: #2, 232-253 February 1970.
10. Levy, W. J. *The current clinical approach to glaucoma.* Rocky Mountain Medical Journal 65: #9, 79-83, September 1968.
11. Richardson, K. T. *The Glaucomas.* Pennsylvania Medicine 72: #5, 61-64, May 1969.
12. Safir, A. and Rogers, S. H. *Ocular effects of juvenile-onset diabetes.* American Journal of Ophthalmology 69: #3, 387-392, March 1970.
13. Shlaifer, A. *A review of glaucoma literature.* American Journal of Optometry and Archives of American Academy of Optometry 47: #1, 3-18, January 1970.

14. Schlaifer, A. *A review of recent literature of glaucoma.* American Journal of Optometry and Archives of American Academy of Optometry 44: #8, 471-489, August 1967.
15. Smith R. J. H. *Clinical glaucoma.* 1965. London, Cassell and Company, Ltd.
16. Stein, J. *Rising incidence of blindness.* MD 12: #1, 93, January 1968.
17. U.S. Department of Health, Education, and Welfare, Public Health Service, *Glaucoma.* Public Health Service Publication #1736, 1968.
18. Veirs, E. R. *So you have glaucoma.* 1958. New York, Grune and Stratton.
19. Virno, M., Bucci, M. G., Pecori-Giraldi, J., and Cantore, G. *Intravenous glycerol-Vitamin C [sodium salt] as osmotic agents to reduce intraocular pressure.* American Journal of Ophthalmology 62: #5, 824-833, November 1966.
20. Virno, M., Bucci, M. G., Pecori-Giraldi, J. and Missiroli, A. *Oral treatment of glaucoma with Vitamin C.* Eye, Ear, Nose and Throat Monthly 46: #2, 1502-1508, December 1967.

7

Is There Hope for the Schizophrenic?

INTRODUCTION

THE ANSWERS TO these five questions are very important to the schizophrenic and his or her family!
   What is it?
   What causes it?
   How common is it?
   What cures it?
   Is there more hope?

WHAT IS IT?

Schizophrenia is a complex illness or group of symptoms and signs which result from the interaction of genetic, metabolic, physical, neurologic, psychologic, sociologic and religious factors. The schizophrenic exhibits many evidences of disturbance in mental function. Frequently, there is no awareness that perceptions through the five senses are distorted. Since these impressions seem real and the schizophrenic acts accordingly, his behavior appears irrational and queer to others. These hallucinations may take place only periodically, however; the person's behavior may be relatively normal at other times. In other words, the schizophrenic speaks a language which we do not understand. He receives impressions which we do not comprehend. His actions are seemingly unpredictable and his moods and expressions of sadness or joy are strange to us. He actually has removed himself from our world and has dropped anchor far away from reality.

Schizophrenia may be defined as an inability to keep the psychologic field organized. This may be revealed as an inability to pay attention to task requirements and a capacity to coordinate messages from various internal systems so that predictable behavior may result.

Although the identification of schizophrenia is frequently difficult, the appearance of symptoms showing a distortion of sense perceptions, thought, judgment, memory and emotions is highly diagnostic.

Do not diagnose yourself but become familiar with some of the warning signs of an approaching schizophrenic episode —*insomnia, headaches, a change in skin color to a darker hue, an ever-present offensive body odor, intense self-preoccupation, irrational crying fits, crippling fatigue, deep depression unrelated to external events, severe inner tension, disturbances in perception, unaccountable changes in personality, inability to lose the feeling of being watched, the growth of a senseless terror, and a fear of loss of self control over one's thoughts and actions.* Some of these symptoms occur in other illnesses but if any combination of them exists, you should immediately consult your physician.

With Doctor Abram Hoffer's permission, Better Health Center (5629 State Road, Cleveland, Ohio 44134), recently published a simple test, the *Symptometer* (a modification of the Hoffer-Osmond Diagnostic Test), for evaluating the presence of such symptoms. It is recommended that the Symptometer be used as a barometer of emotional health. That is, to discover the *danger signs* and to realize the need to see a doctor! A healthy person may score low on this test, but a total score over 30 indicates the need for medical consultation. If it is over 60, one should definitely be under a doctor's care!

SYMPTOMETER

Visual Perception:	*Score*
People's faces sometimes pulsate as I watch them	5
People's face seem to change in size as I watch them	5
When I look at things like tables and chairs, they seem strange	5
My hands or feet sometimes feel far away	5
My hands or feet often look very small now	5
Cars seem to move very quickly now. I can't be sure where they are	5
When I am driving in a car objects and people change shape very quickly. They didn't used to	5
People look as if they were dead now	5
Lately I often get frightened when driving myself in a car	5
People's eyes seem very piercing and frightening	1
People watch me a lot more than they used to	1
People watch me all the time	1
I feel rays of energy upon me	1
Most people have halos [areas of brightness] around their heads	1
Sometimes I have visions of people when I close my eyes	1
Sometimes I have visions of people during the day when my eyes are open	1
Sometimes I have visions of animals or scenes	1
Sometimes I have visions of God or Christ	1
Sometimes the world seems unreal	1
Sometimes I feel very unreal	1
When I look at people they seem strange	1
Often when I look at people they seem to be like someone else	1
Now and then when I look in the mirror my face changes and seems different	1
My body now and then seem to be altered—too big or too small, out of proportion	1
Sometimes the world becomes very bright as I look at it	1
Sometimes the world becomes very dim as I look at it	1
Sometimes when I read, the words begin to look funny—they move around or grow faint	1

Sometimes when I watch TV the picture looks very
strange   1
Sometimes I feel there is a fog or mist shutting me away
from the world   1
Sometimes objects pulsate when I look at them   1
Pictures appear to be alive and to breathe   1
I often see sparks or spots of light floating before me   1
My hands or feet sometimes seem much too large   1
I sometimes feel that I have left my body   1
I get more frightened now when I am driven in a car by
others   1

Auditory Perception:
I often hear or have heard voices talking about or to me   5
I have often heard strange sounds, e.g., laughing which
frightens me   5
I have heard voices coming from radio, television, or tape
recorders talking about me   5
I often hear my thoughts inside my head   5
I often hear my own thoughts outside my head   5
I hear my own thoughts as clearly as if they were a voice   1
My sense of hearing is now more sensitive than it ever
has been   1
I now have more trouble hearing people   1
I often have singing noises in my ears   1
I often hear or have heard voices   1
I have often felt that there was another voice in my head   1

Tactile Perception:
I sometimes feel I am being pinched by unseen things   5
My sense of touch has now become very keen   1
I sometimes have sensations of crawly things under my
skin   1
I sometimes feel rays of electricity shooting through me   1
Some of my organs feel dead   1
I sometimes feel my stomach is dead   1
I sometimes feel my bowels are dead   1
I now have trouble feeling hot or cold things   1
I sometimes feel strange vibrations shivering through me   1
My bones often feel soft   1

Taste Perception:
Some foods which never tasted funny before do so now   1
I can taste bitter things in some foods like poison   1
Foods taste flat and lifeless   1

I have more difficulty tasting foods now   1
Water now has funny tastes   1
Cigarettes taste queer now   1
Olfactory Perception:
Things smell very funny now   5
Other people smell strange   5
Other people's cigarette smoke smells strange—like a gas   1
My body odor is much more noticeable than it once was   1
I sweat much more now than I used to   1
I can no longer smell perfumes as well as I used to   1
Foods smell funny now   1

Time Perception:
I can no longer tell how much time has gone by   5
Time seems to have changed recently, but I am not sure
   how   5
The days seem to go by very slowly   1
Some days move by so quickly it seems only minutes have
   gone by   1
I have much more trouble keeping appointments   1
I have much more trouble getting my work done on time   1
The world has become timeless for me   1
I find that past, present and future seem all muddled up   1

Thought:
There are some people trying to do me harm   5
I can read other people's minds   5
People interfere with my body to harm me   5
People interfere with my mind to harm me   5
I don't like meeting people—you can't trust anyone now   5
Most people hate me   5
I am not sure who I am   5
At times my mind goes blank   1
At times my ideas disappear for a few moments and then
   reappear   1
I am bothered by very disturbing ideas   1
My mind is racing away from me   1
At times I am aware of people talking about me   1
There is some plot against me   1
I have a mission in life given to me by God   1
At times when I come into a new situation, I feel strongly
   the situation is a repeat of one that happened before   1
I now become easily confused   1
I am now much more forgetful   1
I now am sick   1

I cannot make up my mind about things that before did not trouble me	1
My thinking gets all mixed up when I have to act quickly	1
I very often get directions wrong	1
Strange people or places frighten me	1
People are watching me	1
I feel as if I am dead	1
People are often envious of me	1
Many people know that I have a mission in life	1
People interfere with my body to help me	1
People interfere with my mind to help me	1
I know that most people expect a great deal of me	1
More people admire me now than ever before	1

Feelings and Emotions:

I very often am very tired	1
I very often suffer from severe nervous exhaustion	1
I very often have great difficulty falling asleep at night	1
I usually feel alone and sad at a party	1
I usually feel miserable and blue	1
Life seems entirely hopeless	1
I am very painfully shy	1
I am often misunderstood by people	1
I have to be on my guard with friends	1
Very often friends irritate me	1
My family irritates me very much	1
I am often very shaky	1
I am constantly keyed up and jittery	1
Sudden noises make me jump or shake badly	1
I often become scared of sudden movements or noises at night	1

WHAT CAUSES IT?

Since the clinical definition of schizophrenia as an illness or syndrome (symptom complex) continues to be debated among psychiatrists, the problem of establishing causes remains even more elusive. Schizophrenia is an enigma despite much research from many disciplines—genetics, biochemistry, physiology, psychology, sociology, anthropology, epidemiology, psychoanalysis, and clinical psychiatry. Many investigators believe that this disease is the expression of a number of causative factors.

It is increasingly likely that schizophrenia is a symptom complex of disordered thinking, feeling, and behavior rather than a single disease. It also appears that *hereditary, constitutional,* and *environmental* factors contribute in varying proportions to the development of schizophrenic disorders.

The last decade has seen a considerable consolidation of thinking about the cause of schizophrenia. At one time there seemed to be a number of conflicting and antagonistic theories. The *biological* school (organic factors) looked for causes in terms of disturbances of structure-function of the central nervous system. These were said to be inherited or acquired and to act directly on the nervous system, or indirectly through abnormalities of the endocrine (hormone) glands or through disordered metabolism (biochemistry). The *psychological theories* relied on explanations in terms of functional disturbances in thinking and feelings as an end process of environmental experiences. Other theories maintained that *social* influences were most important. These were concerned primarily with direct effects of the human environment at various levels on the learning processes.

It is now evident that these various concepts are complementary and not antagonistic and that no one factor is singly or uniquely at the root of the illness. Thus, schizophrenia is probably the final common path from a number of widely differing etiologic factors. This *multiple causation* was proposed in Chapter Two as a unified concept which applies to the genesis of all disease.

HOW COMMON IS IT?

Psychiatric patients fill approximately one-half of all hospital beds in the nation at any given time. Schizophrenics occupy one-half of these, or 25 per cent of all beds. Data derived from incidence studies lead to the estimate that two per cent of the people born since 1960 will have a schizophrenic experience during their lifetime. Under certain conditions, however, as many as six per cent of them may be so afflicted. It is estimated that nearly one per cent of the entire population of the United States has schizophrenia. Figures vary as to whether two, or five, or ten times as many schizophrenics as are in hospitals live in the community, presenting severe problems for themselves and others. These range from inadequate functioning to endangering the community by acts of a political lunacy or individual transgressions.

Schizophrenia usually strikes early in life and frequently has a crippling effect. Since it occurs mostly in the twenties and thirties, it is said to be more disabling than heart disease or cancer. The average age of all first hospital admissions is thirty to thirty-three years. For other psychiatric admissions, as well as circulatory disease and cancer, the average age is about fifty-one.

On 11 March 1968 an alarming headline appeared in the widely circulated medical newspaper, *Medical Tribune*—"United States Figures Show Mental Illnesses Cost the Public $20 Billion In 1966."

MEDICAL TRIBUNE REPORT
WASHINGTON BUREAU

WASHINGTON, D. C.—Despite improvements in treatment services, mental illness cost U.S. citizens about $20 billion in 1966. Over $9 billion of this amount was borne directly by the public, or an average of nearly $48 for each American, according to figures reported here by Dr. Stanley F. Yolles, director of the National Institute of Mental Health.

A NIMH study of mental illness in 1966 showed that the largest part of the $20 billion—$15.5 billion—was due to decreased productivity of the mentally ill. This includes a loss of $14.3 billion for marketable output, $970,000,000 for homemaking, services, and $240,000,000 for home maintenance and volunteer services.

Treatment and prevention cost almost $4 billion, according to the study. This included more than $2.5 billion spent on in-patient care and more than $1 billion on outpatient care. Patients or their families bore only $500,000,000 of this cost, averaging nearly $200 per patient. Three-quarters of the remainder was expended by local, state, and Federal agencies, with private insurance carriers, private industry, and private philanthropy accounting for the remainder.

These costs were calculated on the basis of the 2,600,000 persons treated for mental or emotional illness in 1966. One-fifth of these or 500,000, were hospitalized on any given day during the year, the report said.

In hospital beds, cost to the economy, and last but not least, personal suffering, schizophrenia can well be considered one of the chief public health problems of this country.

WHAT CURES IT?

Several new methods of therapy have been introduced during recent years. The most important have been custodial treatment and psychotherapy, insulin coma (shock), electric or Metrazol convulsive (shock) therapy, lobotomy (brain surgery), chlorpromazine and reserpine (drugs), and other new agents known collectively as tranquilizers. Estimates of the recovery rates from these treatments range from 18 to 43 per cent.

Treatment	Percentage recovery rate
Lobotomy and supportive treatment	18
Custodial and supportive treatment [psychotherapy]	19
Reserpine	22
Convulsive treatment [electric shock and metrazol]	29
Chlorpromazine	34
Insulin coma [shock]	43

From these data it is obvious that schizophrenia is a serious disease and one for which there is no specific therapy. A recent University of California in Los Angeles Interdepartmental Conference on Schizophrenia summarized the results of treatment in these words:

> We used to think that all schizophrenic patients were inevitably doomed to stay that way. Nowadays I would put it this way: We can expect about one-third of them to go back to pretty good [normal for them] living; we can expect about one-third to be on the borderline; and one-third will not do very well at all.

Where sufficient sums of money for the frequently long and expensive therapy are not available, recovery rates are even more disappointing.

IS THERE MORE HOPE?

The human mind does not exist in a vacuum but is a function of the delicately balanced molecular environment within the brain. Alterations in the concentration of molecular substances which nourish all living cells can greatly alter mental function. An analysis of this theory was recently presented by twice Nobel Prize winner, Professor Linus Pauling, in an article entitled Orthomolecular Psychiatry.

This concept describes the new way in which many investigators and practitioners are looking at emotional disorders. They have found that the identification and correction of biochemical abnormalities in schizophrenics is necessary before further progress is made with the psychological approaches to this problem. In fact, many times the metabolic defects are of such great importance that an almost spontaneous recovery follows their correction. Actually, in the great majority of patients, biochemical or metabolic problems have been noted to be important in preventing recovery.

Many are now seeing that psychoanalysis is not wrong but simply not enough to cure the schizophrenic. An American (H. Osmond, M.D., New Jersey Neuro-Psychiatric Institute, Princeton, New Jersey) and a Canadian (A. Hoffer, M.D., Director of Psychiatric Research, Department of Public Health, University Hospital, Saskatoon, Saskatchewan, Canada) have been treating schizophrenic patients with a megavitamin approach for almost twenty years. Their theory is that megadoses of certain vitamins, Vitamin B₃ in particular, correct the abnormal breakdown of adrenaline (hormone of the adrenal gland) into toxic by-products. These are reported to be the cause of the perceptual alterations in the schizophrenic and the elevated perceptual disorder score (Hoffer-Osmond Diagnostic Test; HOD).

Doctors Hoffer and Osmond have defended their treatment of schizophrenia with controlled research studies:

> We began treating schizophrenic patients with three or more grams per day of nicotinic acid [or nicotinamide] more than a decade ago. We have continued to use this treatment and to study its effect in a series of major therapeutic trials using the full armamentarium of the methodologists; open, single blind and double blind experiments have all been used and their results carefully followed for over ten years. Our findings, based on records which can be inspected and patients most of whom can be easily located, show that when newly admitted schizophrenics are given nicotinic acid treatment of the kind we have used, far more of them remain well than with other treatments presently in use. Our criteria for remaining well or having improved, include —five year cure rates, readmission to a mental hospital, days spent in hospital, clinical status in the community, and the presence or absence of symptoms and signs.
>
> The schizophrenic suicide rate for the patients who did not receive nicotinic acid was 22 times as great as the overall suicide rate. In sharp contrast the rate for patients who were adequately treated with nicotinic acid was near zero, certainly less than the expected community rate.
>
> There can be no a priori reason why massive nicotinic acid should not alter the outcome in schizophrenia. Apart from deep

prejudice or sheer inertia, it is worth trying because it meets one of the major requirements of any treatment, that of 'doing the sick no harm.' Two-thirds of those who develop schizophrenia are more or less crippled by it and return to the hospital for periods ranging from a few weeks to several years. Our studies suggest that at least half of the crippled two-thirds will be well if given nicotinic acid and some of the others will be helped. We think that these young people who are doomed to be in and out of mental hospitals for most of their lives have a right to be given nicotinic acid even if medical men are sceptical. Nothing can be lost and as we have shown, belief or scepticism seems to have very little bearing upon the effects of this treatment.

From accumulated observations of 350 schizophrenics given nicotinic acid (niacin or NAC) or nicotinamide (niacinamide), 3 grams or more daily, and 450 cases without this treatment, Doctors Hoffer and Osmond are convinced that the treatment of choice must include Vitamin B_3. Their ten-year cure rate is now running over 75 per cent compared to only 30 per cent for patients who have not been given the benefit of this simple, safe, and effective chemical. They also have observed no serious toxicities from the use of Vitamin B_3, even for periods of ten to fifteen years.

Extracts from the writings of Doctor Abram Hoffer concerning the method of treating schizophrenia with nicotinic acid (niacin) or nicotinamide were recently printed (with permission of Doctor Hoffer) by the Kirkman Laboratories, Inc. (P. O. Box 3929, Portland, Oregon 97208). Doctor Hoffer classifies his schizophrenic patients into phases and prescribes a treatment approach to each phase. For example, Phase One patients have the best prognosis while Phase Four patients have failed to respond to the other three treatments (Phases One, Two, and Three):

PHASE ONE

These are patients who are ill for the first time or who have relapsed after one or more recoveries by previous treatment. They are able to cooperate with treatment in the community and/or have responsible families who can supervise treatment. The diagnosis is established clinically and the HOD card sort test, Hoffer and Osmond [1961] and the urine mauve test, Hoffer and Osmond [1963] are used for corroboration and for determining the nature of the perceptual disturbances which are present. The patient is informed he has schizophrenia and the nature of the illness is explained. He is advised his chance for recovery is good if he will follow the therapeutic program laid out for him. Following a perceptual hypothesis his symptoms are explained simply as consequences of his illness. He is started on nicotinic acid or nicotinamide at a dose of one gram three times each day. He is seen again in one month. If there has been a substantial improvement, he is continued on the vitamin as an outpatient for one year. After this, the vitamin is stopped, but he is seen and instructed to begin taking the medication again if symptoms return.

Recent research in New York suggests many chronic cases will improve more quickly on doses up to 12 grams per day.

PHASE TWO

These are patients who have not improved adequately on nicotinic acid alone after one month or patients who must be admitted to hospital for treatment. In hospital, they are maintained on the 3 gram dose of vitamin, started on ascorbic acid, 3 grams per day, and given a series of about 6 ECT. Small doses of tranquilizers are used to bring psychotic behavior under control as quickly as possible. If the patients are well seven days after the last ECT, they are discharged. They are then maintained on the vitamin as before for one year as with phase one patients.

PHASE THREE

These are schizophrenic patients who have failed to respond to phase two therapy. They are still in hospital. The vitamin medication is continued as before but in addition they are given penicillamine, 2 grams per day, for about two weeks or until they develop a fever of 103 degrees or a skin rash. They are then given another 3 ECT. As a result of Greiner's [1965] work I am considering the introduction of a low copper diet for phase three treatment.

PHASE FOUR

Phase four patients are schizophrenics who have not recovered after phase three treatment. They become a special research group of great interest. Here a wide variety of treatments are given depending upon the particular diagnosis and problems. These additional treatments include:

(a) The butyrophenones, especially Trifluporidol and Haloperidol. If these compounds are used, 2 mg. of Cogentin per day is given, beginning two days before the butyrophenone.
(b) Thyroid-high doses are given. I increase the dose until the resting pulse rate varies between 100 and 120 per minute, Danziger [1958].
(c) Valium—the patients are given 90 mg. per day for 14 days and then the dose is reduced quickly to 30 mg. per day, Galambos [1964].

OTHER ADDITIONAL TREATMENTS

Everything is done to bring about normal physical health. All foci of infection are treated. If the patient while recovering develops severe anxiety or tension of a neurotic nature, this is controlled with small quantities of barbiturates, Valium or low doses of tranquilizers.

My patients are not given anti-depressants such as aminooxidase inhibitors, sympathomimetic compounds or acetylcholine esterase inhibitors.

Through this period the patients are not given what has been called dynamic therapy. But they are educated about their illness and its symptoms and encouraged to examine their reactions to other people. They are encouraged to pay as little attention as possible to the past and advised they must blame no one for their illness.

RESULTS OF PRESENT PROGRAM

The results will be shown in the following table as recoveries given in percentage of original group.

(*a*) All cases ill less than 2 years.

Phase	Recovered %	Cumulative total %
I	50	50
II	25	75
III	12	87
IV	6	93

This is a conservative estimate. As a comparison, it is necessary to remember that from a similar group not given nicotinic acid, one-third will recover, one-third will revolve from hospital to community, and one-third will not recover. The evidence upon which this statement is based is described in the bibliography.

(*b*) All cases ill over two years.

I have treated 104 cases ill over two years and with an average chronicity of 10 years or more. Out of this 104, 90 patients are well or much improved and are gainfully employed. Only 5 or so are now in any hospital.

TOXICITY OF NICOTINIC ACID AND NICOTINAMIDE

These two forms of the same vitamin are safer than aspirin. It is not possible to commit suicide with them. There are two classes of reactions.

(*a*) Mild but uncomfortable reactions.

These include the flush which comes on when one begins to take nicotinic acid. But, in most cases, the intensity of the flush decreases very quickly with continued medication, until it is hardly more than a gentle reminder that it is still working and active. There may also be a sensation of itching as in sunburn. Young people tend to be more uncomfortable with it. Periactin 4 mg. taken concurrently with nicotinic acid reduces flush a good deal, Robie [1966].

A few people have some nausea which rarely goes on to vomiting. If it occurs, it can be dealt with by stopping all medication and starting very slowly in a few days. One can take a week or so to build up to the full dose.

Also, nicotinic acid produces headache. This can be dealt with by the usual analgesics, and more recently, Adrenaline Methyl Ether in 5 mg. cap. has been very helpful but no company is making it now.

Nicotinamide does not produce a flush and is better for young people. But it may also produce nausea and headache. I usually begin with one and, if the patient is concerned by the reaction, I change to the other.

Nicotinic acid is better for chronic cases and both forms work equally well for early cases.

(*b*) Severe and dangerous reaction.

There are none. In over 350 clinical studies reported in literature, there has been only one case of jaundice. This is less than the expected rate. Another case I know of in New York developed jaundice while taking NAC but was kept on it and his jaundice cleared up. Infectious hepatitis is liable to hit anyone, no matter what medication they are on.

There have been no cases of blood disease or other serious illness. It has been given as a life saving measure to coronary patients, strokes, etc.

Pregnant women have normal babies while on NAC. There is some evidence from animal studies that NAC might have protected women against Thalidomide injured babies.

BIBLIOGRAPHY

Danzinger, L. (1958) Dis. Nerv. Syst. 19, 374-378.

Galambos, M. (1964) Amer. J. Psychiat. 121, 237-274.

Greiner, A. (1965) Personal communication.

Hoffer, A. (1962) I. Newton Kugelmass, M.D., ed., Niacin Therapy in Psychiatry, C. C. Thomas, Springfield, Ill.

Hoffer, A., Mottok, G. and Wilson, D. (1965) Unpublished observations.

Hoffer, A. and Osmond, H. (1952) Report to Dementia Praecox Committee, Scottish Rite Masons, New York.

Hoffer, A. and Osmond, H. (1955) J. Nerv. Ment. Dis. 122, 448-452.

Robie, T. (1966) Report to Int. Assn. A. A. Doctors, Indianapolis.

Hoffer, A. and Osmond, H. (1961) J. Neuropsychiat. 2, 306-330.

Hoffer, A. and Osmond, H. (1964) Acta Psychiat. Scand. 40, 171-209.

A detailed analysis with case reports (for the layman or professional) of the Hoffer-Osmond approach to the treatment of schizophrenia was released by University Books (New Hyde Park, New York) in 1966 under the title, *How to Live With Schizophrenia*. To keep abreast of the rapid advances in the use of Vitamin B$_3$ for schizophrenia and a variety of other disorders, a doctor should secure a copy of *The Vitamin B Therapy; A Second Communication to A.A.'s Physicians* from Bill W., P. O. Box 451, Bedford Hills, New York 10507. Safety, dosage, contra-indications and side effects of B₃ may also be noted in the *Summary* of Chapter Five.

Exciting results from the megavitamin approach to the treatment of schizophrenia have been reported by Doctor David R. Hawkins (M.D.), Director of the North Nassau Mental Health Center, Inc. (1961 Northern Boulevard, Manhasset, Long Island, New York 11030). This is a nonprofit, tax-exempt, voluntary institution which is licensed by the New York State Department of Mental Hygiene and chartered by the New York State Department of Social Welfare. This Mental Health Center specializes in treating schizophrenia, alcoholism, and other perceptual illnesses. It is operated by a professional staff (18 psychiatrists, 2 psychologists, and 2 psychiatric social workers) who are skilled in the use of Vitamin B₃ as a form of chemical therapy for these illnesses.

The North Nassau Mental Health Center is the first, and likely still the only, such facility to evaluate seriously the megavitamin approach in the treatment of schizophrenia. According to Doctor Hawkins, it is clinical results in patients rather than the theory of how or why the vitamins work which is the present primary concern.

In the following report, Doctor Hawkins describes his clinic and evaluates its experience with B₃ therapy during the past four years:

Here are the updated results of our work at the North Nassau Mental Health Center with schizophrenics and alcoholics which were first reported in your 1968 brochure entitled "The Vitamin B Therapy—A Communication to AA Physicians." This summary of our 1968-69 activities makes a total of four years experience with the megavitamin approach to these major illnesses.

My first report to you detailed the treatment effects on 315 schizophrenics, of whom 70 were schizophrenic-alcoholics. These were consecutive cases of patients admitted here during 1966-67. Then for the first time we used massive B-3, which has since become a crucial ingredient in our new treatment program. As a result of the success of this early pilot study our program has since greatly expanded.

In these four years we have treated over 2000 patients—of whom approximately 300 were alcoholics—with the megavitamin approach. Seventy per cent of this large group have exhibited very marked improvement. Most of them could be called recovered; if we define "recovery" as the ability to function satisfactorily in the community with little or no professional help. The alcoholics of course must also be able to maintain their sobriety. Here at the North Nassau Mental Health Center these positive achievements have resulted in the evolution of what can be now seen as a Model Integrated Treatment System with the following ingredients:

1. A treatment center that specializes in schizophrenia, alcoholism and other perceptual illnesses. Our Center is operated by a professional staff who are willing to use chemotherapy featuring the massive use of vitamins, notably B-3.

2. Hospitalization—a facility that accepts referrals with the understanding that our treatment methods will be used. In our case this is a private institution which has become interested enough to conduct research programs of its own and publishes the results.

3. An out-patient clinic which specializes in perceptual disorders and can treat patients in all phases of the illnesses. Our clinic also does clinical research and publishes the results.

4. A half-way house for those who are recovering from the illness or have no home to go to. The orientation of the house is one of rehabilitation in an overall patient regimen compatible with orthomolecular methods (megavitamins, diet, etc.). Weekly meetings of Schizophrenics Anonymous at the house are part of the many activities available.

5. A day care center geared to rehabilitation with an activities program designed for vocation and social rehabilitation.

6. Patient self-help groups including Alcoholics Anonymous and Schizophrenics Anonymous. These are often vital to aftercare in any overall recovery program.

7. Doctors in the community who are skilled in megavitamin therapy and administration of the H.O.D. Test; physicians who will not only treat patients but will be advisors and consultants to such groups as Schizophrenics Anonymous, where continual supervision of medication and diet are so essential.

8. A national organization like the American Schizophrenia Foundation devoted to research, education and the involvement of the patients' families and interested professionals. Here we have the Schizophrenia Foundation of Long Island which fosters

education, family groups, research, fund raising and which backs the Half-Way House and Day Activities Centers.

On Long Island our model is attracting large numbers of schizophrenics and their families. Considerable public interest has also been aroused, and press coverage has been widespread. Many requests for information are coming in, as well as professional visitors from the U.S., Canada and overseas.

The rapidly mounting demand for treatment is reflected in the expansion of our center. We are entering 1970 with a staff composed of 18 psychiatrists, 2 psychologists, 2 psychiatric social workers, 7 secretaries and 5 volunteers. Currently, our outpatient case load is 1200 patients. It is said that our operation has recently become one of the largest of its kind in the greater New York area.

Improved treatment methods have brought some valuable advantages. For examples: The need for hospitalization has been reduced 80 percent. Psychiatric treatment time (per patient) has dropped 80 percent. Out-patient shock treatment is no longer used. The need for extensive psychotherapy has been greatly reduced, and constructive family involvement has greatly increased.

Of course the effect of these developments has been to drastically lower both diagnostic time and treatment costs. Let me illustrate: At most clinics the usual diagnostic procedure is for both family and patient to see a social worker for two separate interviews. This is followed by a diagnostic conference of psychiatrist, psychologist and social worker. The entire process may involve months, during which 12 to 15 hours of professional time has been consumed. This furnishes a diagnosis only; no formal treatment has meanwhile been possible.

By contrast, our current procedure requires only the "HOD" diagnostic test plus a single interview with a psychiatrist. In 90 percent of our cases, this gives us a definitive diagnosis at a nominal cost. Because this can be done so quickly, we save both family and patient that endless waiting before treatment can start.

The total treatment time is also greatly reduced. We see the average patient 15 times the first year, and 4 to 6 times the second year. It should be borne in mind that in most cases we are treating severely ill people, many of them having multiple problems, as well as schizophrenia.

Our approach continues to move in the direction of searching for certain biochemical abnormalities in patients and correcting these first, before we commence to deal with any psychological approaches to clinical problems. We have found that the great majority of our patients to have biochemical and metabolic problems, conditions which have been extremely important in preventing any worthwhile recovery. In a very sizable percentage of patients, once these abnormalities are corrected rapid progress and recovery is the usual outcome.

Alterations of the molecular concentration of the substances normally present in the human body can greatly alter mental functioning. This important concept was convincingly presented by Nobel prize winner Dr. Linus Pauling in 1968, in an article entitled "Orthomolecular Psychiatry," *Science,* April 19, 1968. To many of us now working in this field, Dr. Pauling's concept very accurately describes the approach that we have been actually using for the past four years; an approach based on the extensive original work of Drs. Hoffer and Osmond that began in 1952.

Our clinic also treats alcoholic patients. Among them three problems appeared over and over again which were either responsible for slips, or prevented full emotional recovery despite sustained sobriety. The first problem we check is the use of the hypnotics, barbiturates or the so-called minor tranquilizers. The effect of taking even small amounts of these substances seriously interfere with the patient's sobriety and brings about subtle alterations in his thinking and feeling, and sometimes outright slips. In *every single case* where these medications have been used, the effect was noticeably deleterious.

Functional hypoglycemia (hyper-insulinism), or so-called low blood sugar, was another factor commonly present and previously undetected. This condition accounted for many failures to recover. Such alcoholic patients immediately felt better as soon as they were taken off sugar and sweets and placed on B-3 to elevate their blood sugar levels. We found this marked improvement to be as clinically conclusive as obtaining a five-hour glucose tolerance test in the laboratory.

Of the alcoholics who did get the five-hour glucose tolerance test many reported that during the testing they began to develop symptoms which they recognized they had often experienced periodically, and which often preceded drinking. Quite a few patients who had been sober for considerable lengths of time reported periodic depressions, feelings of tension, anxiety and recurrent desires to drink. Correction of the hypoglycemia eliminated these symptoms in the great majority.

The third problem we discovered in alcoholics, which played a very important part in delaying or preventing recovery, was the presence of multiple perceptual distortions as revealed by administering the HOD test.*

This is a test for alterations of perceptions such as touch, taste, hearing, vision and perception of bodily parts with associated feelings. There are also alterations in the perception of time and space which show up on the "HOD." These malfunctions have a profound effect on mood, judgment and the ability to discriminate reality.

Most alcoholics who have just sobered up will show a high HOD score initially. But this rating rapidly returns to normal following continued sobriety. However, in many of the patients we see, who are unable to get sober, or who are sober but still miserable, an elevated HOD score persists. Such changes in perception are thought to be due to alterations in brain function on a chemical basis, due perhaps to abnormalities of adrenalin metabolism as described by Drs. Hoffer, Osmond, and many others. In some patients the HOD score was so high as to give the alcoholic symptoms of schizophrenia, so that it was difficult to say whether the patient had schizophrenia complicated by alcoholism, or alcoholism which had developed into schizophrenia. Though hallucinations are common during DTs, many such alcoholics continue to have hallucinations long after they have stopped drinking. The great majority of our group also had functional hypoglycemia, and they, too, were emotionally and mentally quite ill. Although these perceptual problems appear to occur more often in the younger alcoholics, we nevertheless screen every alcoholic patient with the HOD test.

All these patients responded very well to a combination of Vitamin B-3 in doses of four grams or more per day; ascorbic acid four grams per day, with the addition of 50 mgs. a day of pyridoxine. In many cases Vitamin E, 200 international unit capsules, four times a day were added. Many patients who are on niacin report a greatly diminished desire to drink as well as alleviation of other symptoms.

The theory behind the megavitamin approach is that the megavitamins correct the abnormal breakdown of the adrenalin into toxic byproducts which are the cause of the perceptual alter-

---

*See Bill W's 1968 *Communication to AA Physicians*—"The Hoffer-Osmond Diagnostic Test for Schizophrenia." (HOD Test equipment available at Bell Therapeutic Supplies, Inc., 382 Schenck Avenue, Brooklyn, N.Y. 11207.)

ations and the elevated HOD score. Practically speaking, when we take patients off harmful drugs, correct their hypoglycemia and then place them on megavitamins, sometimes with the addition of one of the phenothizine drugs, remarkable recoveries are often the result. It is clinical results rather than theory which concern us at the present time.

Within the last year, a new chapter of Schizophrenics Anonymous started on Long Island. Many AA's who have rather marked perceptual distortions identify with both SA and AA. In fact, many of the SA groups recently formed in the United States and Canada have been started by AAs who had perceptual problems. (The growth and success of these SA groups was reported in World Medical News in a special article on Schizophrenics Anonymous in December 1969.) Quite a few alcoholics have entered AA after SA had first helped them to correct their perceptual problems. Only then were they able to recognize and deal with their alcoholism.

The SA groups have all located doctors in their several communities knowledgeable about the megavitamin approach or who are truly interested in learning how to work with it. The number of doctors utilizing the megavitamin therapy is now proliferating at such a rate that the finding of suitable medical assistance should no longer be too difficult. The national headquarters of A.S.F. has an expanding referral list of such physicians.*

DAVID R. HAWKINS, M.D., *Director***
North Nassau Mental Health Center, Inc.
1691 Northern Boulevard
Manhasset, Long Island 11030

CASE REPORTS

Approximately 70 per cent of the patients treated during the past four years at the North Nassau Mental Health

---

*American Schizophrenia Foundation, 610 S. Forest Avenue, Suite 6, Ann Arbor, Michigan 48104.

**Dr. Hawkins is editing the first book on Orthomolecular Psychiatry which will be published in 1970 entitled *Orthomolecular Psychiatry: Treatment of Schizophrenia*. This edition will include contributions by twenty-three different authors and will include a chapter on Schizophrenics Anonymous, the first sizable patient group to make use of this new approach in helping to solve their problems.

Center have shown a very marked improvement. In fact, most of these could be called *recovered* according to Doctor Hawkins. To illustrate this dramatic breakthrough in therapy, he briefly describes five patients:

Case One: I refer to this case as my "Lobotomy, Yes—Niacin, No!" case. This patient is a 33-year-old housewife and mother of four young children. She had been ill for an indefinite period but overtly and severely psychotic with schizophrenia for five years. The family had unlimited means and left no stone unturned in providing the best of professional help. She was in a number of hospitals and was treated by a number of highly qualified psychiatrists. In addition to this, she had all the psychotropic drugs in massive doses and in multiple combinations, as well as several courses of electroshock therapy. Despite all this, her condition became progressively worse. She was openly delusional, suicidal, homicidal, out of contact and violent. Because of the hopelessness and severity of her condition, the physicians and hospital finally recommended a prefrontal lobotomy (in 1968 this was an almost unheard of procedure, as the results are often rather grave and irreversible which indicates the extraordinary severity of her condition.)

The patient was scheduled for the lobotomy and at the last minute, the family asked if she could be given a trial megavitamin therapy before resorting to the drastic surgery procedure. At this point, the psychiatrist in charge of the case became infuriated at the family's temerity and exclaimed—"Lobotomy, yes—Niacin, no!" The family then had the patient transferred, against medical advice, out of the hospital and had her admitted to Brunswick Hospital in Amityville, Long Island. The patient was not at all happy about the transfer, did not like the new hospital, did not feel the new treatment would help her, did not like her new doctor, but *did* consent to take medications.

On a combination of megavitamins, thyroid, hypoglycemic diet and a small dose of tranquilizers she recovered in 10 weeks. She was discharged from the hospital 14 months ago and during the intervening time has returned to full normalcy, including taking care of her children, running her household, becoming active in PTA and other social activities and she is now working at a half-time job in addition. When interviewed currently, she gives no noticeable signs of ever having been ill, and she is being seen for after-care for about twenty minutes every 10 weeks. She looks well, feels well and has no symptoms.

Case Two: A 45-year-old man who had been sick continually for 10 years and had been given up as hopeless after many hospitalizations, years of therapy, all the drugs, shock treatments, insulin coma therapy, etc. His diagnosis was that of chronic paranoid schizophrenia, and the doctors had advised committing him for the rest of his life. The family, however, could not bear this prospect and so had kept him at home for several years where his condition was so incredible as to sound like a horror story out of a Victorian novel. He screamed obscenities out the window at his hallucinatory enemies, refused to shave, bathe, get a haircut, or change clothes and threw new clothing out the windows when it was offered. He refused to take any medication and eating was sporadic and bizarre. He was unable to function in any capacity, had no interest, even in TV. There was no way of reaching him and the family came to the clinic on his behalf. The family refused recommitment, so that the only treatment approach feasible was to put the megavitamins surreptitiously in his food. Together we worked out a concoction of niacin and ascorbic acid powder mixed with bicarbonate of soda and mixed with a little chicory to cover the flavor in his coffee (he was a big coffee drinker). We saw the family every two or three months to check on his condition, and by the end of a year he had made such progress that he was now a clothes dandy, ate normally, was able to remember, was no longer hallucinating, now watched TV, carried on a normal conversation, read a daily paper, was calm, and, according to the family and neighbors, the extent of his recovery was unbelievable. He is currently looking for a job and to this day, because he still refuses to take any kind of a pill, he is unaware that he is getting large doses of megavitamins.

Case Three: This case concerns both schizophrenia of childhood onset and severe drug involvement over a number of years. This 23-year-old young man was a behavior problem since early childhood and had been in continuous treatment since the sixth grade when he had become quite disturbed. The family had made considerable sacrifices and had him as well as themselves in treatment with some very famous and highly qualified psychiatrists. Despite this, the patient's condition worsened, and he became heavily involved in the drug scene where he became addicted to barbiturates and amphetamines and in addition took LSD, STP, hashish, marijuana, demerol, dilaudid, opium, kief, hog, cocaine, mescaline, psilocybin, THC, Freon, amylnitrate, morphine, dexamyl, carbona, etc. and heroin. He lived on the streets in New York City, and his condition was disheveled, malnourished and bizarre. He shot methedrine intravenously and had a $140-a-day consumption of speed so that, in addition, he also developed needle hepatitis. The family managed to bring him in just once for a diagnostic evaluation and, at that time, his HOD score was over 100. He then disappeared back into the city and showed up a number of months later in an acute drug crisis at Bellevue Hospital where he had been taken by the police (Speed plus STP).

He was transferred to the Brunswick Hospital in Amityville where his clinical course was extremely stormy. He was uncooperative, disturbed and hallucinating, and, in addition, had generalized jaundice with markedly abnormal laboratory tests. With intensive treatment in the hospital, he was discharged in 8 weeks but still had an intense craving for methedrine. Although out of the hospital, he was unable to function in any way, was very regressed and did nothing but watch TV.

During the ensuing year, he has been on megavitamins, plus large doses of Vitamin B-3 and small doses of tranquilizers. It is now 14 months since he was discharged from the hospital, and his HOD score is now 8, indicating the disappearance of any active schizophrenia. The craving for drugs has disappeared, and he, in fact, now counsels young people who are currently in trouble with drugs. He is working full time, active in community affairs, is involved with a very normal young woman and is now moving on to a responsible job involving administrative responsibility in the counseling of young people who are still quite ill due to drugs plus schizophrenia.

Case Four: A 28-year-old single, young man who had been ill for six years. He had been treated by all known methods, including drugs, electroshock therapy, etc., and had spent the last four years at one of the highest priced famous psychoanalytically oriented, private psychiatric hospitals in the United States. While there, he received almost daily psychoanalytic sessions but became worse and worse to the point that he had stopped eating and the family feared for his life. The institution refused to use any drugs and, instead, used wetpacks, restraints, seclusion. The institution even refused to give him an injection so that he could be transferred and, instead, sent him up to Brunswick Hospital tied up in wet sheets and restraints. His arrival presented an almost unbelievable sight, and the patient admitted frankly he was committing suicide by starvation because he could not bear the agony of his illness any longer.

This patient was so ill that we had to institute electroshock therapy treatments, but in 10 weeks he was discharged on a combination of megavitamins, plus phenothiazine drugs. He very shortly returned to work and during the last two years has done very well with an active social life as well as a responsible work record. We see him every 8 weeks for about 20 minutes to check on his medication and to see how he is doing. His family spent close to *$200,000* on his previous treatment up to the time that he arrived here in mummy fashion.

Case Five: This is a 34-year old alcoholic and schizophrenic who had had a long, unsuccessful history of treatment with many hospitalizations, shock treatments, arrests and ultimate total rejection by his family. His alcoholism took a florid and bizarre trend. When drunk, he became assaultive, had blackouts, smashed up cars, got into violent fights, and he was totally unemployable. In addition, he had delusions and hallucinations even when he was not drinking and felt so depressed that he had to return to drinking. He had tried AA but was too ill to comprehend the program.

He never dated and felt he was homosexual, as he had a number of homosexual experiences. In addition to all the other troubles, he was addicted to a combination of Doriden, Librium, Valium, and, occasionally, amphetamines, which he took to keep from passing out from the combination of other drugs (he averaged over 40 pills a day). He was unsuccessful in getting off this combination of drugs because of either severe withdrawal or convulsions. We withdrew him from the addicting drugs as an out-patient and switched him to heavy doses of non-addictive phenothiazine tranquilizers. He was taken off sugar and sweets because of his hypoglycemia and placed on heavy doses of megavitamins. In addition, he went to Schizophrenics Anonymous. Within several months, the schizophrenia symptoms abated, although the drinking continued. Finally, he became sufficiently rational to follow the suggestion that he give AA as well as Schizophrenics Anonymous a chance, and his drinking stopped abruptly.

By the time he celebrated his first anniversary in AA he was working, was off Welfare, was going to dances and learning how to socialize. During the second year, he received a promotion, then went on to a better job, became engaged, and at the end of the second year married a very nice girl. During the third year, they had the first baby whom they bring with them when they come to the clinic which is now two or three times a year. He is still active in AA as well as SA and has helped a great many other ill people recover.

HYPOGLYCEMIA

Reports from research psychiatrists and clinicians who use the megavitamin approach have pointed out that many emotionally ill patients, including schizophrenics, have broad fluctuations in blood sugar (or glucose). They note that recovery is not complete in many until this metabolic flaw is corrected. Doctor Harry M. Salzer (M.D.) of Cincinnati, Ohio, has observed that this defect is one of the most common causes of neuropsychiatric illness and occurs in 30-40 per cent of his private patients. He has proposed that it be called relative hypoglycemia and defined it as "a clinical syndrome in which patients develop symptoms referrable to any system of the body as the result of a relative drop in blood sugar level in response to a high carbohydrate food intake and drinks containing caffeine." In the past this syndrome has been called functional hyperinsulinism, essential hypoglycemia, functional hypoglycemia, dysinsulinism, hypoglycemic fatigue, and neurogenic hypoglycemia. Doctor Salzer has found that a drop of 20 milligrams or more below the fasting blood sugar level during a six-hour glucose tolerance test is sufficient to make a diagnosis of relative hypoglycemia of non-organic origin, and can produce many neuropsychiatric symptoms.

Relative hypoglycemia mimics any neuropsychiatric disorder, and such patients have been diagnosed as having psychoneurotic anxiety, psychoneurotic depression, depressive reactions, schizophrenia, manic-depressive psychosis, psychopathic personality, chronic alcoholism, convulsive disorders, migraine, idiopathic cephalalgia, second cervical root syndrome, neurodermatitis, and even hypertensive cardiovascular disease.

According to Doctor Salzer, the major symptoms may be

classified as psychiatric, neurologic or somatic. In 300 private patients with relative hypoglycemia he has observed these symptoms in the following percentages of this group:

PSYCHIATRIC SYMPTOMS

Depression	60%
Insomnia	50
Anxiety	50
Irritability	45
Crying spells	32
Phobias	31
Lack of concentration	30
Forgetfulness or confusion	26
Unsocial or antisocial behavior	22
Restlessness	20
Previous psychosis	12
Suicidal	10

SOMATIC SYMPTOMS

Exhaustion or fatigue	67%
Sweating	41
Tachycardia	37
Anorexia	32
Chronic indigestion or bloating	29
Cold hands or feet	26
Joint pains	23
Obesity	19
Abdominal spasm	16

NEUROLOGIC SYMPTOMS

Headache	45%
Dizziness	42
Tremor [inward or external]	38
Muscles pains and backache	33
Numbness	29
Blurred vision	24
Muscle pains and backache	33
Staggering	18
Fainting or blackouts	14
Convulsions	4

Doctor Salzer's prescription for these 300 patients with relative hypoglycemia was: (1) a diet high in protein and fat and low in carbohydrate, (2) nutriment between meals and every two hours throughout the evening, (3) abstinence from any medication or beverage containing caffeine, and (4) 6-12 ten cc. intragluteal injections of calcium-glycerophosphate.

By following the corrective diet and receiving the injections, approximately 85 per cent of these patients either recovered or were greatly improved. Parenthetic mention should be made that these 300 patients had been to other physicians, had been treated with sedatives and tranquilizers, and even electro-convulsive therapy, without showing improvement. Some had even been on a corrective diet without improving because the diet was not followed closely (Doctor Salzer's Hypoglycemia Diet suggestions can be found in Chapter Five: Is There Hope For the Alcoholic?)

Salzer makes a plea for the six-hour glucose tolerance test as a routine procedure for psychiatric or neurologic evaluation. He says that the correction of relative hypoglycemia can spare a patient years of agony:

> By making the diagnosis of relative hypoglycemia and teaching patients what they should eat, they will be spared years of suffering, electro-shock therapy, and the hazards inherent in taking sedatives, stimulants, and tranquilizers.

SUMMARY

There is a remarkable new hope for the schizophrenic. Nutritional therapy has been shown to produce extraordinary improvement and recovery in many patients.

The restriction of dietary carbohydrate, an increase in protein and unsaturated fat, and the utilization of megadoses of Vitamin B_3 and Vitamin C, in addition to psychotherapy, have the potential for revolutionizing schizophrenia treatment.

From the evidence presented, it appears that sugar and other highly processed carbohydrates are detrimental to the schizophrenic and that vitamins, minerals and protein are beneficial. Hence, based on the earlier definitions (Chapter Two), these carbohydrates must be viewed as susceptibility factors in schizophrenia. Conversely, protein, vitamins and minerals may be regarded as resistance agents.

To find out more about the nutritional treatment of schizophrenia, one may write—The American Schizophrenia Foundation, 610 S. Forest Avenue, Suite 6, Ann Arbor, Michigan 48104, or The American Schizophrenia Association, 56 West 45th Street, New York, New York 10036.

REFERENCES

1. American Schizophrenia Foundation. *What you should know about schizophrenia.* 1965.
2. Bellak, L. and Loeb, L. *The schizophrenic syndrome.* 1969. New York, Grune and Stratton.
3. Better Health Center, 5629 State Road, Cleveland, Ohio 44134, *Megavitamin therapy.* Seventh edition. June 1969.
4. Bleuler, M. *The genesis and nature of schizophrenia.* Psychiatry Digest 30: #1, 17-26, January 1969.
5. Dunham, H. W. *Community and schizophrenia; an epidemiologic analysis.* 1965. Detroit, Wayne State University Press.
6. Grinker, R. R. *An essay on schizophrenia and science.* Archives of General Psychiatry 20: #1, 1-24, January 1969.
7. Harrison, T. R., Adams, R. D., Bennett, I. L., Resnik, W. H., Thorn, G. W., and Wintrobe, M. M. *Principles of internal medicine.* Fifth edition. 1966. New York, McGraw-Hill Book Company.
8. Hoch, P. H. and Zubin, J. *Psychopathology of schizophrenia.* 1966. New York, Grune and Stratton.
9. Hoffer, A. *Enzymology of hallucinogens.* pages 43-55, *Enzymes in mental health.* G. J. Martin and B. Kisch [authors]. 1966. Philadelphia, J. B. Lippincott Company.

10. Hoffer, A. *Niacin therapy in psychiatry.* 1962. Springfield, Illinois, Charles C. Thomas.
11. Hoffer, A. *Treatment of schizophrenia with nicotinic acid or nicotinamide.* October 1965. Kirkman Laboratories, Inc., P. O. Box 3929, Portland, Oregon 97208.
12. Hoffer, A. and Osmond, H. *Treatment of schizophrenia with nicotinic acid.* Acta Psychiatrica Scandinavica 40: #2, 171-189, 1964.
13. Medical Tribune Report, Washington Bureau. *U. S. figures show mental illnesses cost the public $20 billion in 1966.* Medical Tribune and Medical News 9: #21, 3, March 11, 1968.
14. Salzer, H. M. *Relative hypoglycemia as a cause of neuropsychiatric illness.* Journal of the National Medical Association 58: #1, 12-17, January 1966.
15. Smythies, J. R. and Antum, F. *The biochemistry of psychosis.* Scottish Medical Journal 15: #1, 34-40, January 1970.
16. Smythies, J. R., Coppen, A., and Kreitman, N. *Biological psychiatry.* 1968. New York, Springer-Verlag, Inc.
17. The UCLA Interdepartmental Conference. *Schizophrenia.* Annals of Internal Medicine 70: #1, 107-125, January 1969.

Are There Any Other Hopes?

INTRODUCTION

THE EMPHASIS THUS far has been hope for a number of relatively incurable disease syndromes. Obviously, there are many others—too many in fact to be included in this book. Additionally, there are medical problems which cannot be rightly considered to be a specific disease state but rather a puzzling mechanism of disease which heretofore has defied explanation and treatment. This chapter will briefly concern itself with some of these incurable disorders and several mystifying mechanisms which are presently considered incurable.

WHAT ABOUT CANCER?

No one needs to be reminded of the commonness of cancer and its far too frequent devastating end results. One of the most frequent forms of cancer in the female is that which involves the cervix (neck) of the uterus (womb). It is generally held that the overall average cancer cure rate, despite improvements in detection and refinements in treatment, is about fifty per cent.

This cancer, like many others, is classified into various groups or stages, based upon the degree of malignancy. For example, for this kind of cancer, the classification ranges from stage 1 (the least malignant) to stage 4 (the most vicious). When success is viewed in terms of the degree of malignancy, the average five-year percentage survival rates approximate 75, 50, 25, and 5, respectively. Thus, viewing the salvage percentages in terms of those living at the end of five years, there is unquestionably ample room for improvement.

At the present time, there are two forms of therapy for cervical cancer. One is surgical; the other radiation. The former is usually employed when there is reasonable evidence that the entire cancer mass can be successfully cut out. In the event that this is not deemed possible, radiation is the treatment of choice. However, many advocate radiation in early cervical cancer. Obviously, in situations where surgery is performed and there is still some question as to whether all the tumor has been extirpated, radiation is also used. Radiation is designed to accomplish two ends. First, it exerts a direct damaging effect upon the tumor cells. Second, the indirect effect upon the tumor is mediated through its action on the host and the tumor bed. Successful radiotherapy (as the procedure is called) is the product of the direct and the indirect influences upon the cancer.

One of the big questions for many years has been: how to develop a method of determining whether all of the cancer has been eliminated? Rosa Graham, a celebrated cancer cytologist at the Roswell Park Hospital for Cancer in New York, noticed back in 1947 that, following radiation treatment, the cellular configurations observed in a vaginal smear could be correlated with the cancer prognosis. The technique was named the Radiation Response, usually referred to as the RR. Without becoming involved in the intricacies of the technique, suffice it to say that the RR is expressed by a number ranging from zero to 100. The higher the number, the greater the indication that all of the cancer has been eliminated. It is generally recognized that 70 or higher represents a favorable response.

Apropos, we at the University of Alabama Medical Center conducted a study with 54 female subjects with biopsy-proven squamous cell carcinoma of the uterine cervix. One group of 27 women received the usual radiation treatment for cancer. A like group, paired by age and cancer stage was provided wlth dietary counsel in addition to radiation. Specifically, one week prior to the initiation of radiation, a nutritional regime was instituted and continued during and for three weeks after radiation.

Mention should be made that in earlier chapters, refined or highly processed carbohydrates were observed to be a *susceptibility* factor in a number of disorders. Hence, the elimination of these foods was designed to minimize the possible host susceptibility to disease. Earlier evidence in this book demonstrated the fact that protein, vitamins, and minerals serve as *resistance* factors. It was for this reason that these nutrients were encouraged.

Each subject was instructed to consume a relatively high-protein low-refined-carbohydrate diet. Animal protein (meat, fish, and fowl) was encouraged at each meal. Carbohydrates of low nutritional value (desserts, sweet snacks of all kinds, sugar) were virtually eliminated. This dietary regime was selected for two reasons. First, because it provides an optimal intake of protein, vitamins, and minerals. Second, a seven-day dietary record taken from these patients indicated that, as a group, they were consuming a relatively high-refined-carbohydrate low-protein diet. In addition, multivitamin-trace mineral supplements were provided in therapeutic amounts.

Approximately three weeks following the termination of the radiation treatment, the RR was assessed in both the control and the experimental groups.

In the control category, those women receiving only the traditional radiation therapy without supplementation, the RR scores ranged from zero to 100. Hence, this suggests, first and foremost, that the response to radiation was quite variable. In this group, the average RR was 63. If a desirable RR is 70 or higher, then, as a group, the control patients fared badly. Actually six out of ten displayed a good RR. Put another way, forty per cent of these women did poorly.

In the experimental series, characterized by nutritional support as well as radiation, the RR scores ranged from a low of 91 to a high of 100 with an average of 98. Hence, in every instance, on the basis of 70 as the delineating point, this group did well.

From these preliminary observations, and they must be viewed as just a pilot study, four items warrant reemphasis. First, in routine cases with radiation alone, the Radiation Response is quite variable. Second, the average response to radiation leaves much to be desired. Third, simple dietary correction and supplementation yields decided change in the Radiation Response. Lastly, the experimental group shows a decidedly good prognosis.

If one may assume that there is a correlation between radio-curability and radiation response (RR), then it would follow that the experimental group characterized by radiation with dietary change should fare better than the control series both in terms of morbidity and mortality. Our observations with these groups over a period of several years suggest that this is true.

There is an increasing interest in the possibility of parallelisms between cancer and the modern diet. For example, Doctor Denis P. Burkitt, a noted British surgeon and epidemiologist, discussed this subject in San Diego at the American Cancer Society's National Conference on Cancer of the Colon and Rectum.

Part of his thesis is that refined carbohydrates, such as sugar and white flour, play a major part in the pathogenesis of cancer of the bowel and colon.

The exciting question which immediately comes to mind is the mechanism by which the radiation response is altered by dietary means. The answer, at this date, is not forthcoming. However, there is abundant circumstantial information to suggest interesting possibilities. For example, it is well known that diet influences the hormonal system. The scientific literature is replete with data which show that diet is an important ingredient in many enzyme systems which are vital to body metabolism. Much has been written about hormones and cancer; much is known about cancer and enzymes. Possibly all of these areas are related.

It would seem, from these limited observations, that there may be more hope for the cancer patient by nutritional means!

WHAT ABOUT HEART DISEASE?

Heart disease is the number one killer of our time. There are obviously many different kinds of heart disease. The type which is most common and most disabling results from a lack of blood to the heart muscle itself. All cells and tissues of the body must have blood, and the heart must pump it out to all organs. But the heart *itself* requires blood. For our purposes here, suffice it to say that the coronary blood vessels are the route by which the heart receives its own nourishment through its own blood supply.

With time, these vessels may become hardened and thickened, and the passage through them narrows. This leads to increasingly less blood delivered to the heart muscle. Also (and not uncommonly), a blood clot may lodge in one of these heart vessels and cut off the blood supply entirely in a matter of seconds to part of the heart.

There are many ways of approaching almost any kind of a problem or situation. For example, one can examine a house for its esthetic quality, or its electrification, or its plumbing. Similarly, there are many different techniques available for assessing the extent of heart damage. One such tool is the electrocardiogram. The electrocardiogram is nothing more than a graphic representation of the electrical activity which precedes the muscular action of the heart. Here again, there are several views which one can examine much as one can study the esthetics of a home in terms of its color, shape, size, etc. In the case of the electrocardiogram, different aspects are analyzed by attaching wires to the arms and a leg. The reading obtained from the two arms is somewhat different than the picture derived from one arm and one leg. Whatever the method, the end result is a pictorial pattern describing a number of waves and segments. Approximately 13 different measurements in millimeters and milliseconds can be derived from a single electrocardiographic tracing.

One of the highly diagnostic features of the standard electrocardiogram is the so-called T wave. In scientific terms it represents the wave of repolarization through the vital ventricles of the heart. Simply, it expresses one feature of the electrical ripple in its passage through the ventricles—the muscular masses of the lower chambers which are charged with the responsibility of propelling the blood throughout the body and through the lungs.

The height of the T wave, expressed in millimeters, has been carefully studied in health and disease. It is generally conceded that, with advancing age, the height of the T wave progressively declines. Thus, for example, at one point in time, it may be two millimeters high. Later in life, the height may only be one millimeter. This same change, though more abruptly, occurs in the case of certain types of heart attack. Hence the T wave, as well as other electrocardiographic parameters, is used as one measure of heart muscle damage.

The height of the T wave has been investigated in health, with aging, and in many disease states. It is also of interest for predictive purposes. Insurance companies are particularly interested in this electrocardiographic indicator because it is prognosticative of heart disease. For example, in allegedly healthy individuals, the height of the T wave has been shown to correlate with future mortality. The lower the height, the greater the mortality risk.

With this information as background, we took 42 presumably healthy dental students in their early twenties. Twenty-one were given glucose solutions and 21 received a low-calorie artificially sweetened drink. Electrocardiograms were taken on all subjects on Monday (prior to the supplements) and Friday (after three days of the supplements) of the same week.

The most exciting observation was the fact that the height of the T wave decreased in the group of students supplied the glucose supplement for only three days. This did not occur in the controls receiving the low-calorie drink. These data parallel the scientific literature which shows that highly processed (refined) carbohydrate consumption can markedly and unfavorably modify the pattern of the T wave. The obvious practical conclusion to be drawn from these admittedly limited data is that a reduction in sugar and sugar products should be desirable since it would tend to protect the individual against this unfavorable reflection of heart status. This is quite consistent with earlier analyses in this book showing that sugar and other highly processed carbohydrates are *susceptibility* factors in a variety of diseases.

Thus, it would seem, within the limits of these simple observations, that there is more hope, mediated through relatively simple dietary means, for the patient with potential heart disease!

WHAT ABOUT CONGENITAL DEFECTS?

It is a curious fact that we, in the Western World, have traditionally held to the view that the really important part of life commences when we are born. For example, for this reason, we calculate age from the day of birth. In contrast, the Chinese have long appreciated the importance of prenatal time; age is counted from the day of conception. By our attitude, we have neglected a period in the history of man which is without doubt most important to his subsequent development and his anticipated three score and ten years.

The developing human spends about 266 days in the womb. He starts out as a fertilized egg the size of one-fourth of that of a period at the end of a sentence, weighing approximately one twenty-millionth of an ounce. Within a matter of nine months, the baby must present itself to the world about twenty inches in length and seven pounds in weight. Thus, from conception to birth, weight must increase about two billion times!

The true extent of congenital malformations is really not known. However, estimates are available. For example, at the Columbia Presbyterian Hospital in New York City, congenital malformations have been identified in approximately seven per cent of live-born infants. Surely, some born dead also have congenital defects. Some malformations may be so subtle as to only make their clinical appearance later in life or possibly not at all. The National Foundation tells us that, in the United States, 250,000 infants are born each year with significant birth defects. The point is that, by all estimates, congenital malformations are very common.

In order to understand the genesis of congenital defects, it is necessary to have some idea of the terms used to describe this developing creature. The period of the *ovum* refers to the interval from conception to the end of the second week. The term *embryo* is applied to the organism from the end of the second week to the end of the eighth week. The designation *fetus* refers to the period beginning with the ninth week until the time of birth. Obviously, these are rather arbitrary periods since development proceeds gradually from one to another during the nine-month gestation period.

There is no question but that infants are born with defects which can be ascribed to genetic factors. It is estimated that this represents about ten per cent of all malformations. At the present time, there is very little that can be done to resolve the problem. Our concern here must necessarily be exclusively with the factors which influence the intrauterine environment. Once these are recognized, steps can be taken which would conceivably reduce the large number of youngsters born with congenital defects.

If one were asked to pinpoint the most important period in intrauterine development, the answer must unequivocally be the first twelve weeks. This is so because within this early period the fundamental cells are formed, and from them the basic tissues are developed so that the organs have begun to take shape. This should not be interpreted to mean that the remaining twenty-six weeks are unimportant. However, the complexities in the fetal period are not as significant as basic design, and this occurs early in gestation.

The point should be underscored here that many and diverse factors may influence the child's development. Surely, all of us have read of the relationship of German measles to congenital malformations. One large area which offers some hope for congenital defects is the problem of nutrition and its effect upon the developing baby.

Perhaps the most classic and terrifying demonstration in recent times is the action of thalidomide upon malformations. It is now thought that the mechanism by which thalidomide exerted its harmful effect was that it interfered with the metabolism of Vitamin B$_6$, also called pyridoxine. Apparently, this vitamin deficiency at a crucial time in intrauterine development was enough to produce horrible malformations (e.g. missing limbs). The developing organism is highly sensitive to change in its environment. For example, a particular vitamin shortage for a matter of two or three hours at a special time in development can be enough to seriously scar a lower animal. Applied to humans (if this be possible), a vitamin or other deficiency for two or three weeks could possibly be the basis for a congenitally defective child.

There are a number of experiments in scientific literature which are relevant to this discussion. For example, Peer and his co-workers at the Saint Barnabas Medical Center in Newark carried out a program with 594 pregnant women who had previously given birth to a child with a deformity (including cleft lip and/or cleft palate). Of this group 418 women did not receive vitamin therapy during a subsequent pregnancy. Another 176 women were supplied with a vitamin regime during the first three months of pregnancy. Among the children born to the 418 untreated mothers, about 8 per cent had various deformities and of this group 5 per cent had a cleft lip and/or cleft palate. In contrast, in the group of 176 vitamin-treated women who gave birth, approximately 3 per cent had deformities of one type or another with only two per cent showing cleft lip and/or cleft palate defects. Much still remains to be explored in this field. One must wonder what would have happened had the dosage been increased or extended or started earlier. It is interesting to speculate about the results if other nutrients besides vitamins had been introduced. Notwithstanding, it is exciting that, in this simple experiment, there was about a fifty per cent decline in malformations when the vitamin-treated subjects were compared with the control series.

This is noteworthy since earlier discussion of a variety of disorders has shown vitamins consistently to be a resistance factor in disease.

These data would suggest that there may indeed be more hope for the prevention of some of the terrifying congenital defect problems!

Mention has been made that there are isolated but interesting and possibly significant relationships between congenital defects and many environmental factors. The instance of the virus of German measles was briefly cited. More immediately, the exciting observations in New Jersey with vitamin supplementation were mentioned.

Many other penetrating experiences have also been reported in medical circles. For example, Navarette and his colleagues in Mexico studied the incidence of congenital defects as they relate to sugar metabolism. Specifically, these investigators performed the glucose tolerance test. This is a procedure whereby one measures the blood sugar levels over a period of time (e.g. every half hour for three hours) after subjecting the patient to an oral or intravenous load of glucose and possibly other agents (e.g., cortisone). They observed a prevalence of abnormal glucose tolerance tests of about 58 per cent in patients who had previously delivered a malformed infant. This was in sharp contrast to 3 per cent abnormal glucose tolerance tests in a sample of women who delivered children without such defects. Hence, they conclude the possibility of a relationship between abnormal sugar metabolism and congenital defects. The observations here are consistent with earlier evidence that sugar is a *susceptibility* factor in disease. Parenthetic mention should be made that the B-complex vitamins are known to influence favorably sugar metabolism.

Once again, here is some evidence that there may be more hope for the prevention of the congenital defect!

WHAT ABOUT MENTAL RETARDATION?

Doctor George Tarjan, Superintendent and Medical Director, Pacific State Hospital (Pomona, California) and Associate Professor, Department of Psychiatry, University of California School of Medicine in Los Angeles, sets out for us quite clearly the multifactorial nature of this devastating problem and identifies for us its method of measurement:

> There is general agreement that mental retardation is a syndrome which can be caused by many factors acting singly or in combination. . . . In practice, we use significant impairments in two aspects of behavior—intelligence and general adaptation—as the guideposts of diagnosis.

How common is it? The late Doctor Abraham Levinson, Professor of Pediatrics at Northwestern University Medical School in Chicago and his staff quote the following appalling figures on the incidence of mental subnormality:

> In 1946, the American Association on Mental Deficiency estimated that 7% of the population is mentally or intellectually deficient. Of 13,000,000 men examined for Selective Service up to 1944, 4.3% were rejected because of mental deficiency. . . . The figures given for the incidence of mental retardation in children vary. Dr. Charlotte Graves states that there are an estimated 10 million exceptional children in the United States or 25% of the child population under 18 years of age. Other authorities believe that there are 5,000,000 retarded children in the United States, or 12.5% of the child population.

It really matters little which figures one accepts. The simple fact is that mental deficiency is a big problem in the United States.

Scores and scores of scientific publications have already appeared showing that intelligence and intellectual behavior can be substantially improved in all kinds of lower animals by simple nutritional means. There is a dearth of material relating to humans. For example, there are data in print demonstrating an improvement in mentation with orange juice, thiamin, riboflavin, niacin, iron, lecithin, and Vitamin E.

One group of investigators headed by Ruth F. Harrell of the Department of Psychology and Education at the College of William and Mary in Williamsburg, Virginia, has dramatically shown the effect of prenatal vitamin supplementation upon the intelligence of the offspring. One group of women was supplied with vitamins during pregnancy, and another group was given pills indistinguishable from the vitamins but containing no nutrients (placebo). The study is especially noteworthy because the vitamins were not given until relatively late in pregnancy. Nothing was done to the children after birth. At the age of three or four it was noted that the intelligence quotients of the children whose mothers received vitamins were substantially higher than the scores in the children whose mothers did not receive vitamins. In fact, the difference was about 8 per cent. The importance of this difference is heightened by the following quote from Doctor Joaquin Cravioto (Associate Director, Institute of Nutrition of Central America and Panama):

> In an increasingly complicated world of sophisticated technology in which even a mild reduction in mental performance may be a serious handicap, the possible effect of early malnutrition on mental capacity and personality development should be a major consideration.

In short, here is one more instance of a possible hope for a seemingly incurable problem!

SUMMARY

Presumably how many and how much hope there is for incurable disease is in large measure a matter of definition. To the patient with a disease for which no solution has been given, a glimmer is a lot of hope. How incurable is incurable and what may rightly be called curable also determine the answer to the question.

Surely, there are, to say the least, thousands of Americans

who have headaches which do not respond to traditional medical therapy. To an individual with recurrent, stubborn headaches, this is an incurable problem. The fact that an aspirin will lessen or abolish the headache for a variable period of time does not disqualify this type of headache from the realm of incurable diseases.

With these definitions of what constitutes hope and what is incurable, presented in this chapter are some short but exciting subjects. We see that there is more hope for cancer. We learn of new avenues to solving heart disease. We discover that dreaded congenital problems can be aborted. There is even more hope for the mental retardate!

Doctor Burkitt summarizes the thinking of many investigators with this statement:

> Evasive action can be taken long before the actual causative agents are understood. Cholera was evaded by the avoidance of sewerage—contaminated water a century before the Vibrio Cholera was identified as the cause of the disease.

REFERENCES

1. Burkitt, P. P. *Modern diet may play role in cancer of the bowel.* J.A.M.A. (Medical News) 215, #5, 717, 722, February 1, 1971.
2. Cheraskin, E. Ringsdorf, W. M. Jr., Hutchins, K., Setyaadmadja, A. T. S. H., and Wideman, G. L. *Effect of diet upon radiation response in cervical carcinoma of the uterus.* Acta Cytologica 12: #6, 433-438, December 1968.
3. Cheraskin, E., Ringsdorf, W. M., Jr., Setyaadmadja, A. T. S. H., and Barrett, R. A. *Effect of carbohydrate supplements upon the height of the T wave in Lead I.* Angiology 19: #4, 225-231, April 1968.
4. Craviota, J. *Application of newer knowledge of nutrition on physical and mental growth and development.* American Journal of Public Health 53: #11, 1803-1809, November 1963.

5. Harrell, R. F., Woodyard, E. R., and Gates, A. I. *The influence of vitamin supplementation of the diets of pregnant and lactating women on the intelligence of their offspring.* Metabolism 5: #5, 555-562, September 1956.
6. Levinson, A. and Bigler, J. A. *Mental retardation in infants and children.* 1960. Chicago, The Year Book Publishers.
7. Montague, M. F. A. *Prenatal influences.* 1962. Springfield, Charles C. Thomas.
8. Navarette, V. N., Torres, I. H., Rivera, I. R., Shor, V. P., and Garcia, P. M. *Maternal carbohydrate disorder and congenital malformations.* Diabetes 16: #2, 127-130, February 1967.
9. Peer, L. A., Gordon H. W. and Bernhard, W. G. *Effect of vitamins on human teratology.* Plastic and Reconstructive Surgery 34: #4, 358-362, October 1964.
10. Tarjan, G. *The next decade: expectations from the biological sciences.* Journal of the American Medical Association 191: #3, 160-163, January 18, 1965.

9

Can We Stay Young?

INTRODUCTION

THE THEME THROUGHOUT the book thus far has been that there is indeed some hope for the incurable. The discussions have led us to consider diverse problems like multiple sclerosis, the alcoholic, the patient with progressive and refractory glaucoma, the schizophrenic, and other afflictions which are presently held to be incurable. We have not only learned that there is some hope but that the aforementioned syndromes are relatively common. After all, about nine million Americans suffer with alcoholism, roughly two million with glaucoma, approximately two million with schizophrenia, and so forth. So, in the aggregate, incurable problems afflict a sizable segment of the American public.

But not a word has been uttered about the most common of the incurable problems, namely, the aging process. While getting old is inevitable, it *can* be slowed so that, in the words of the celebrated Doctor Paul Dudley White, more life can be added to our years rather than simply adding more years to life!

It would, therefore, be well to ask ourselves the very same questions about the aging phenomenon which have been raised in earlier chapters.

What is it?
What causes it?
How common is it?

What cures it?

Is there more hope?

WHAT IS AGING?

Scientific literature is replete with data about age, aging, and the aged. According to Doctor Bernard L. Strehler, Professor of Biology at the University of Southern California Gerontology Center, there are ten myths about growing old which have barred us from taking the needed steps to increase the human life span. These ten myths were recently discussed at a conference on aging at the Center for the Study of Democratic Institutions in Santa Barbara, California.

The first and foremost of the myths is that man, in some unknown fashion, has the capacity to achieve physical immortality. It was a dream of this sort that began Ponce de Leon's search for the fountain of youth. This illusion is the basis for many present-day fads and fancies, injections, and rest cures. Unfortunately, the simple fact of the matter is that evolution has made immortality a fairy tale. Biologically, man consists of trillions of cells. Some of these units have been programmed to grow and mature in a particular fashion. These cells and their tissues cannot be replaced. Their deterioration is inevitable, and death must follow.

A second myth is that man cannot extend the Biblical three score and ten. No other primate lives as long as man. No other animal takes so long to mature. It seems logical that, if evolution has allowed man to live longer than any other primate, further progress is well within the realm of probability. Doctor Strehler adds, "It would be even more naive to think the rate of aging can't be modified by environmental factors like diet, drugs, and selection of long-lived progenitors."

A third myth is the belief that longer living is just science fiction. The proponents of this fable admit that longer life is perhaps possible, but not in the very near future. But laboratory animals have shown that life *can* be extended. If one can extrapolate from these studies to man, the consensus is that man's life can be extended fifteen to twenty-five years in people presently living. There are even people living today who are beyond 100 years of age and are enjoying good health. In lower animal research, for example, there are chemicals which slow cellular oxidation. Scientists are of the opinion that this approach can be applied to humans. Even relatively simple observations lead us to believe that longevity can be extended in the very near future. For example, Doctor Benjamin Berg has extended the life of certain small animals from their usual 280 days to about 500 days by caloric restriction alone. This type of information is almost immediately relevant to humans, since obesity in man is known to shorten life expectancy.

A fourth myth contends that slowing or decline and postponement of death would create greater economic burdens on society. However, this fantasy ignores the fact that longer life cannot be accomplished without improving general health. Put another way, if senility is delayed, then the bothersome aspects of senility are likewise postponed!

Myth number five suggests that longer-lived people will multiply social problems because older people are more conservative and, therefore, obstruct social change. The counter-argument is based upon the fact that this assumption ignores the probability that socioeconomic attitudes are more a function of the *kind* of life one leads and not *how long* one actually lives. For example, equal housing for blacks is more opposed in white lower-middle class communities than it is in suburban retired neighborhoods!

The sixth myth is that longer living would increase the problems of the population explosion. This whimsy pays no attention to the fundamental factor which limits the quality of life—the individual's ability to produce goods and provide services. Clearly, longer and more active lives would increase productivity.

Number seven in the myth series is that we should not tinker with the life span because this is interfering with nature. In other words, if God wished us to live longer, we *would* be living longer. This argument ranks with the one that if God meant for us to fly, He would have given us wings!

Number eight is the proposition that aging has an intrinsic charm and wisdom which is not possible without getting old. The counter-argument is that elderly persons derive their values from their experience, and not from their deterioration!

Perhaps the most devastating of the myths, item nine, is that prolonging life will mean surrounding the environment with decrepit, unsightly, depressed, and dependent people. As is the case with some of the other notions, it pays no attention to the fact that one cannot prolong life without improving health.

The last of the myths is the most defeating. It contends that present-day research is sufficient and that progress with regard to longevity is adequate. The simple fact of the matter is that about fifteen million dollars a year is spent on this particular problem. This would not even buy every American man, woman, and child a chocolate bar!

If one investigates the appearance of any of the classical disease states, it becomes evident that with advancing years more and more people become afflicted. As the population grows older, there is progressively more cancer, heart disease, arthritis, blindness, and so on. Even without considering the classical syndromes, it is a fact that, with advancing age, the blood pressure progressively rises, the serum glucose slowly climbs, performance slows, there is memory loss, the skin wrinkles, teeth are lost, and sexual drive diminishes. It is an undisputed fact that people show the ravages of age. It is *normal* to age—if one grants that normal is defined as *average*.

But the other question which must be answered is whether it is *healthy* to age. The fact that normal (average) and physiologic (healthy) are not synonymous is an obvious clinical fact. Who has not encountered a person who is chronologically thirty but looks sixty and behaves and complains as if he were sixty? Conversely, is it not a fact that someone else may be chronologically sixty and look and act and behave as though he were in his thirties? The fact that there is anyone in this world who is ninety and behaves like fifty proves at least one point. Namely, it is *possible* to live to be ninety chronologically but be *physiologically* fifty.

There is no one definition of aging and aged. The most humorous and possibly the most accurate definition is that anybody ten years older than you are is old. If this does nothing else, it emphasizes the relativity of aging. Aging, like life, cannot be defined. It can, however, be described, and that has been done extensively in our scientific literature.

Scientists have analyzed tens and possibly hundreds of physiologic functions. For example, comparisons have been made between the functions of man at the age of thirty (calling this 100 per cent) and again at seventy-five. It is noteworthy that brain weight is almost halved. The number of filtering tubes in the kidney (glomeruli) is cut in half. Almost two-thirds of the taste buds on the tongue vanish. The hand grip is half as good. These and scores of other measurements have provided the characteristics for normal (average) aging at a particular age. But the question is whether these parameters may be regarded as being physiologic (healthy) at the same age.

WHAT CAUSES IT?

The only point about aging more difficult to define than what it is, is what causes it. There are bushels of theories about the cause of aging. One of the glaring reasons for the mass of hypotheses is that each is evolved to serve a specific purpose by an investigator with a particular viewpoint. For example, aging can be viewed from a chemical, physical, psychological, economic, etc., point of view. The answer is obviously dependent on the viewpoint.

For our purposes, the aging theories may be classed into *three* broad categories. First, there are very *general* theories. Second, there are what might be called *intermediate* theories. Finally, there is a set of *basic* theories.

The general theories indicate that aging is due to one of several possibilities. For example, there is the notion that the aging process is the result of depletion of irreplacable material as a result of sheer living. Another hypothesis simply indicates that mortality is inversely related to vitality. As vitality diminishes, mortality increases. A third ill-defined concept is that there is a converging of a disturbance in a number of physiologic variables which lead, in some obscure way, to aging. A more current general theory is that aging is a result of an accumulation of life stresses and the consequent damage of such stresses. Lastly, one philosophic thesis is that aging is an adaptive phenomenon designed to increase the survival of the species by eliminating the older members of the group.

Whatever merits these general hypotheses may have from a philosophic standpoint, they do not really come to grips with the underlying chemistry necessary to explain the aging process. And these theories are impractical because they do not provide suggestions on how aging may be slowed, or even reversed.

The second group of theories may be viewed as the intermediate type. Within this category, there are a number that should be mentioned. One very popular hypothesis is that aging is simply the result of the progressive decrease in the number of cells in the body. A more recent thesis, the "cybernetic" theory, points out that there is a slowing down of the transmission rate of impulses through the nervous system, and this results in a lack of coordination which finally disorganizes the human organism beyond repair. This is a very interesting explanation. However, it does not provide an answer as to how aging causes the slowing of impulses through the nervous system.

As one might expect, there is one theory that explains aging on the basis of hormonal imbalance. There is no question that, in some instances, the administration of hormones may indeed slow or break the aging process. However, the unresolved question is still *why* hormone-producing glands tend to decline in activity with time. The theory that enzyme deterioration is a major factor in the aging process is also a very interesting hypothesis. It is well established that the content of most, though not all, cellular and tissue enzymes decreases with age. This can, unquestionably, be an intermediate cause of many of the changes which occur with time. But the question again is *why* there is enzyme deterioration. There is no doubt that one of the important mechanisms in the aging syndrome relates to auto-immunity. It suggests that, with the progression of age, very large molecules emerge or are so altered that they are no longer recognized by the system's immunologic defences, and they are then attacked by the person's own body. The theory of somatic mutations states that cellular distortions cause the development of inferior cells and tissues. Another hypothesis is that aging is the result of continuous radiation damage. One theory stresses the importance of toxins (poisons) which develop in the digestive tract with advancing time.

All of these hypotheses are of interest. However, they can

only be regarded as intermediate theories because they do not describe why the changes that are held to be causative do indeed occur.

The third group of theories may be viewed as basic. Within this category there are a number one finds interesting. The "clinker" theory holds that, with age, there is the accumulation of waste particles within the cell. These particles are physiologically inactive and, in a sense, throw a wrench into the works. The protein hysteresis theory contends that, with time, there is coagulation of protein materials. The thermal denaturation theory supposes that irreplacable molecules are rendered nonfunctional by thermal inactivation. There is a calcification-calciphylaxis theory. This concept holds that uncontrolled deposits of calcium are the cause of many of the symptoms and signs of aging. Possibly the most talked-about explanation currently in circulation is referred to as the cross-linkage theory. This hypothesis contends that large molecules which are necessary for life processes are progressively immobilized within the cells and the tissues by the linkage of various elements inside the cell. This renders the cells inactive. Cell death, according to this hypothesis, can be caused particularly by cross-linkage of DNA which is the vital protein molecule within the cell nucleus.

In brief, it can be safely said that, even in the light of the basic theories, there is no generally accepted chemical cause or explanation for the aging process. However, as we shall see, there are reasonable observations suggesting that it may very well be possible to prolong life.

HOW COMMON IS IT?

Clearly, unlike the other problems mentioned in earlier chapters, aging is inevitable. In this regard, therefore, the incidence is 100 per cent! However, what is more important is that some people seem to age faster than others. All of us have been surprised, some time or other, to learn an individual's age because he seemed to be much older or younger than his years.

WHAT CURES IT?

As we have learned from earlier discussions in this chapter, it is generally held that aging is inevitable and, it must follow, incurable. However, it is clear from the evidence of lower animal studies that senility can be delayed. The general theories mentioned earlier contribute nothing to the problem. The intermediate theories are perhaps more fruitful. The cross-linkage and clinker theories seems to be the most tenable ones, for they center on the initiating stage of the aging syndrome. Hence, it provides a logical point of attack for prevention and possible reversal.

For practical reasons, the central question is whether it is possible to reduce the level of cross-linkage with diet. The cross-linking agents are numerous and involve so many essential life processes that it is difficult to identify a particular nutrient. However, there is evidence in lower animals to indicate that an overall caloric reduction avoids the accumulation of cross-linking compounds. Thus, the restriction of food seems to prolong life quite clearly in several lower animal species.

There is some limited evidence that an adequate level of Vitamins C and E will slow, if not reverse, the aging process in certain lower animal groups.

IS THERE MORE HOPE?

The eminent nutrition authority, Doctor Roger J. Williams (Professor of Biochemistry at the University of Texas) asserts that many of the infirmities and diseases of aging could be substantially slowed down, if not entirely avoided by proper nutrition. In other words, through nutritional improvement, aging individuals can live out their lives relatively free from disabling disease.

A recent editorial in *Geriatric Focus* magazine expressed Doctor Williams' view in this fashion:

> Enumerating various changes characteristic of aging [impaired vision, hearing, memory, strength, and endurance; insomnia; loss of libido and appetite for food; aches and pains; increased tendency toward constipation, arthritis, diabetes, arteriosclerosis, osteoporosis, senility, etc.], he said: "I want to call attention to the idea that every one of these signs of old age probably is connected with failure of the cells and tissues somewhere in the body to perform their functions properly; and also that every one of these failures is related to cell and tissue nutrition. . . .
>
> "Without concerning ourselves with the problem of whether there is an irreversible aging process in all cells that cannot be overcome, we can state with assurance that the longer cells are furnished with the necessities of life, including good nutrition, the longer they will continue to remain in good working order."

We would agree with Doctor Williams that the answer to this question, *Is There More Hope?,* is an unequivocal yes!

There are isolated scientific studies suggesting that it is possible to modify the inevitable aging process. Some of these will be considered at this time.

It should be recalled that there is no universally accepted definition of aging. Additionally, it should be evident that there is no universally acceptable cause for the aging process. However, certain inescapable facts cannot be ignored. It is clear that, with aging, there are increasingly more symptoms and signs. It is obvious that elderly people with more complaints are more apt to die. It is certain that individuals with more complaints are not as healthy as those with fewer or no complaints. Hence, it is fair to make the assumption that, all other factors being equal, individuals without complaints are in better health than those with complaints, and that individuals without complaints are more apt to live longer than persons with complaints. In a sense then, the fewer complaints, the younger the individual!

For the past five years, we have been conducting a health evaluation project of 433 doctors and their wives. One group is centered in Tampa, Florida, a second contingent in Los Angeles, California, and a third center in Columbus, Ohio. It should be emphasized that the observations stemming from these three areas are very similar. This suggests that the data is reasonably representative. Earlier consideration (Chapter Three) has been given to some of the dietary habits of these individuals.

Many parameters of health and disease were studied in these families. One such was the number of complaints described by each participant. This was accomplished by requesting that each subject complete the Cornell Medical Index Health Questionnaire. This is a very simple self-administered form of 195 questions, to be answered yes or no. The questions are so structured that a positive reply suggests a medical problem. Hence, by simply counting up the number of affirmative responses, one has a crude index of the patient's health status. By this technique it was learned at the initial examination of this group that there were approximately 17 complaints per subject.

At the initial session, a dietary record was obtained. The method of dietary analysis may be of interest to the reader and, accordingly, will be outlined in Chapter Ten. The dietary results were presented to the group so that each participant could see first hand his or her own eating patterns. Lectures were then offered to emphasize the merits and the shortcomings in their dietary habits. This information will be discussed in some detail in the next chapter.

One year later each member of the group completed the Cornell Medical Index Questionnaire for the second time, and the dietary record was taken. It was then possible to compare the clinical responses over a one-year period. It is noteworthy that the average number of complaints for the entire group dropped to 12. In other words, within the one-year period, the clinical picture of the group improved approximately 30 per cent. Specifically, the average fifty-year-old doctor had, at the start of the project, about 20 positive responses in contrast to 19 yes answers in the 40 year age group. After studying their own dietary patterns and in many instances altering them, the fifty-year-old male revealed a mean number of 15 complaints. Thus, in fact, this older group became more like the 40-year-old group within twelve months. In a sense, it appears that it is possible to reverse the clinical process of aging.

It is most exciting to consider the possibility of diminishing, rather than increasing, complaints as we get older. Particularly thrilling is the potential of accomplishing this goal by relatively simple dietary means. However, the evidence should be viewed with caution. One serious limitation is the method of obtaining the data. The questionnaire technique always invites the risk of inaccuracy. Second, there is no control group for comparison. For these and other reasons, it might be appropriate to look at the doctors and their wives from another vantage point.

It is now generally known that certain blood chemical tests can be used as predictors of specific disease states. For example, much has been published in the scientific journals about the coronary proneness profile designed to anticipate the occurrence of a heart attack. Part of the profile depends upon measurements of the fat content of the blood. This is usually done by calculating the cholesterol and/or triglycerides in blood serum. The higher these values are, the greater the risk for heart disease.

These tests were performed in the group of practitioners and their wives. Brief consideration will be given here to the serum triglyceride scores as representative of the problem. First, it should be pointed out that, under physiologic conditions, serum triglyceride levels should be between 50 and 150 milligrams per cent. At the initial visit the average serum triglyceride score was 193 milligrams per cent. If one grants that the upper acceptable border is 150, then 193 is about one-third higher than it should be, and the risk for heart disease is obviously greater. Following lectures describing the condition and dietary alterations which could be instituted, the serum triglyceride level for the group dropped to 110. Thus, within about a one-year period, by means of relatively simple dietary changes in some of the group being observed, the average serum triglyceride level had returned to within the relative no-risk zone. In effect, the blood level had been cut almost in half! On the assumption that people with relatively higher serum triglyceride levels are more apt to become clinically ill, then it is fair to conclude that this group has been made younger in terms of this particular aspect of the aging process. In a sense, the findings pictured here at the biochemical level parallel and, therefore, support the data earlier outlined at the clinical level.

One instance of braking the aging process at the *clinical* level has been described. One example at the *biochemical* level has been offered. Now, as a final illustration, let us glance at the *physiologic* level.

The electrocardiogram is a graphic representation of the electrical activity which precedes the muscular activity of the heart. Just as one can view a house from different angles (the front, back, top, bottom), so one can examine the heart's activity from different aspects. Wires (called leads) are attached to different parts of the body and to a recording device. The most common connections consist of the two arms and one leg. By turning a switch on the machine, one can obtain a record from, let us say, the two arms. This is called Lead I.

The end-result, the electrocardiogram, consists of a series of waves which can be measured up and down, in the vertical (in millimeters) and in the horizontal axis (in milliseconds). Actually, in Lead I, it is possible to quantitate thirteen different characteristics of heart activity. For example, one little bump on the electrocardiogram is called the P wave. Its height (in millimeters) and duration (in milliseconds) can be measured with reasonable precision. This P wave is a reflection of the wave of electrical activity (called depolarization) in the atria (upper chambers) of the heart. The QRS complex is another area which can be measured. It, for our purposes here, signifies the wave of electrical activity through the ventricles (lower chambers) of the heart. The P-R interval (measured in milliseconds) is an index of the time required for the impulse to start in the pacemaker of the heart and pass through the atria and become ready to fire the ventricles.

It is well known in scientific circles that with advancing age the P-R interval lengthens. In fact, when one compares this particular electrocardiographic parameter in infancy and again in elderly people, the difference is found to be about 70 per cent longer in the old group. Hence, because this is commonly observed, it is said to be normal. If one grants that normal means average, then it is truly normal for the P-R interval to lengthen slowly with time. However, there are older people who show a P-R interval not unlike a young person. The question then arises as to whether this is good or bad. If it is normal (average), with age, to show lengthening of the P-R interval, then is the old person with a young P-R interval ill? In other words, is normal (average) synonymous with physiologic (healthy)? Surely, it is normal (average) to have dental decay since 95 per cent of Americans have dental decay. However, it is generally agreed that it is physiologic (healthy) to have no decay. It would therefore appear that, while it is normal (average) to show lengthening of the P-R interval with time, it is physiologic (healthy) to show little or no lengthening of the P-R interval with time.

The P-R interval was studied in the group of doctors and their wives. It was found that, with advancing age, the wave did indeed lengthen in this group just as it does in people in general. The electrocardiogram was restudied subsequent to lectures on diet as previously outlined. Interestingly enough, in each age group, the P-R interval became shorter. Specifically, by example, in the oldest age category (60+ years), the average P-R interval at the start of the study was 0.169 seconds; at the end of the study, 0.157 seconds. Noteworthy is the fact that the mean P-R interval of the 45-60 year age group prior to dietary instruction was 0.158 seconds. Hence, within this one year experimental period, the 60+ year old subject became like the 45-60 year old was at the beginning.

In simple terms, by simple dietary means, it is actually possible to reverse the process and demonstrate the fact that people can be made younger at heart!

SUMMARY

All about us there is evidence that the aging process can be slowed or hastened in plants and lower animals. For example, the sea anemone can be maintained for over 80 years with absolutely no evidence of becoming old. Tadpoles can grow new tails and earthworms new parts without any difficulty.

Even in humans, there is some proof, though admittedly incomplete. Children may be born with *progeria*. At birth there may already be all of the peripheral signs of a very old individual. By the age of ten or fifteen years of age, the skin is wrinkled, the hair is totally gray or white, there is hardening of the arteries and other characteristics of a sixty or seventy-year-old person.

There are obviously many unanswered questions and much research to be done. But even viewing the problem in its most simple and practical form, there seems to be immediate hope for the aging if one accepts certain propositions. First, older persons are greater risks for sickness and death. Second, older individuals have more complaints, more pathologic biochemical patterns, more electrocardiographic aberrations, etc., than younger folks. Third, older subjects with more complaints, poorer biochemical state, more pathologic electrocardiograms represent a greater morbidity and mortality risk than older persons with relatively fewer complaints, better biochemical and electrocardiographic state. Granting these qualifications, it is noteworthy that members of the health profession and their wives show a reversal to a better clinical, biochemical, and electrocardiographic pattern following simple dietary counsel. A resounding yes. It would appear that there is some hope for the aging process!

REFERENCES

1. Bakerman, S. *Aging life processes.* 1969. Springfield, Charles C. Thomas.
2. Battista, O. A. *The timely challenge of research on aging.* The Chemist 46: #2, 67-72, February 1969.
3. Cheraskin, E. and Ringsdorf, W. M., Jr. *Clinical findings before and after dietary counsel.* Geriatrics [pending publication]
4. Cheraskin, E. and Ringsdorf, W. M., Jr. *Serum triglyceride levels before and after dietary counsel.* [submitted for publication]
5. Cheraskin, E. and Ringsdorf, W. M., Jr. *Younger at heart: a study of the P-R interval.* Journal of the American Geriatrics Society 19: #3, 271-275, March 1971.

6. Editorial: *Slight excess of vitamins is recommended for aged.* Geriatric Focus 9: #2, 9-10, February 1970.
7. Getze, G. *Expert's view: mythology of aging thwarts longer lives.* Los Angeles Times, April 21, 1970.
8. Novosti Press Agency. *Very old people in the USSR.* The Gerontologist 10: #2, 151-152, Summer 1970.
9. Riley, M. W. and Foner, A. *Aging and society: volume one: an inventory of research findings.* 1968. New York, Russell Sage Foundation.
10. Shock, N. W. *The physiology of aging.* Scientific American 206: #1, 100-110, January 1962.
11. Tappel, A. L. *Where old age begins.* Nutrition Today 2: #4, 2-7, December 1967.
12. Tappel, A. L. *Will antioxidant nutrients slow aging processes?* Geriatrics 23: #10, 97-105, October 1968.
13. Walker, A. R. P. *Can expectation of life in Western populations be increased by changes in diet and manner of life?* South African Medical Journal 43: #25, 768-755, June 21, 1969 [Part Two].

10

Does Diet Offer Hope of Preventing Incurable Diseases?

INTRODUCTION

IT IS APPARENT from mortality and morbidity figures that chronic disease is rampant in the United States today (Chapter One). These data show both a true increase now and a greater increment projected for the years to come. Since the current annual bill for health care is sixty-one billion dollars, it is imperative that disease causation be more adequately understood so that prevention of disease can be more effective.

Numerous factors are responsible for causing a particular disorder, even an acute infection (Chapter Two). Although the environment (germs, viruses, etc.) plays an important role, it cannot fully explain disease causation. For disease to occur, environmental factors must act upon a body (host) which, for various reasons, has an increased susceptibility and/or a decreased resistance. The science of medicine, if not the practice of medicine, now knows some of the ingredients of host state (resistance and susceptibility). Included in this group is diet.

There is reason to believe that two dietary problems exist in the United States. One of these, *undernutrition,* is largely the result of poverty. The other, *malnutrition,* may exist in any household. It is the outcome of poor food selection and dietary ignorance. According to recent national surveys of dietary patterns, it is clear that significant nutrient deficits exist (Chapter Three).

One point which should be underlined is that sugar and highly processed carbohydrate products furnish approximately one-fourth to one-third of the total calories ingested. This is of significance for three reasons: (1) these foods are protein, vitamin, and mineral poor; (2) their utilization by the body requires large quantities of vitamins and minerals which, literally, have to be stolen from other foods or body tissues; (3) they replace foods, such as meat, vegetables and fruits, that are rich in protein, vitamins and minerals. This combination of deficits is a glaring example of malnutrition in the United States. Malnourishment from these nutrient-poor carbohydrate calories is a principal contributor to America's number one nutritional problem—obesity (overweight).

Adding to this burden is the fact that we live in a culture where a considerable decrease in the nutrient content of food occurs between the garden and the gullet (Chapter Three).

Although there is much to be learned about the disorders discussed in Chapters Four through Nine, considerable hope has been observed with nutritional therapy. The regimes recommended included the following:

1. Restriction of dietary carbohydrate, especially sugar, syrup, and very highly processed starch foods.
2. Restriction of saturation fats and replacement with the unsaturated fats.
3. Multiple vitamin-mineral supplementation.
4. Megadoses of Vitamin C and Vitamin B.

Parenthetic mention should be made that Items 1 and 2 may meet the requirements stated on p. 16 ff. for a *susceptibility* factor. Also, Items 3 and 4 appear to qualify as *resistance* factors (see p. 16 ff.).

From this discussion it becomes apparent that nutritional

regimes which aid in recovery from multiple sclerosis, alcoholism, glaucoma, schizophrenia, heart disease, cancer, and aging are similar to that needed for improvement of the average American's diet. It is likely that the diets offering more hope for the incurable may also prevent the development of these disorders or delay their onset to the autumnal years. Such a preventive diet might be termed The Optimal Diet.

What are the features of such a regime?

NUTRIENT NEEDS

Recommended Dietary Allowances: Since 1940 the Food and Nutrition Board of the National Research Council has formulated standards of dietary adequacy for the human residing in the United States. Pertinent scientific information and research are periodically reviewed. On the basis of such analyses, judgments are made regarding which nutrients and in what amounts are necessary for the maintenance of good nutrition of practically all healthy people subjected to the usual everyday stresses. The original recommendations have been reconsidered six times, the most recent revision being in 1968. The RDA (Recommended Dietary Allowances) should not be confused with the MDR (Minimum Daily Requirements) of specific nutrients prepared by the United States Food and Drug Administration (FDA). The Minimum Daily Requirements are those below which demonstrable deficiency signs, presumably, occur. They are used primarily in labeling foods. The RDA serve a very different purpose:

> Excepting calories, the allowances are designed to afford a margin sufficiently above average physiological requirements to cover variations among practically all individuals in the general population. The allowances provide a buffer against increased needs during common stresses and permit full realization of

growth and reproductive potential, but they are not necessarily adequate to meet the additional requirements of persons depleted by disease, traumatic stresses, or prior dietary inadequacies.

The Recommended Dietary Allowances, Seventh Revised Edition (1968) for ages ten to seventy plus are listed in four tables (see end of chapter). The allowance levels are intended to cover individual variations among most *normal* (average) persons as they live in the United States under *usual* environmental stresses. Previous revisions of the RDA have been made without any radical departures from the initial pattern of nutrient formulations. However, in the 1968 revision, a number of important changes have been instituted. These are summarized in a table (see end of chapter). In addition to the new nutrients for which specific allowances were established, the following micronutrients were discussed as essential or possibly essential: Vitamin K, choline, biotin, pantothenic acid, copper, fluorine, chromium, cobalt, manganese, molybdenum, selenium, and zinc. The need for the electrolytes (sodium, potassium, and chloride) and water were also considered. The recommended reduction in calories was basically a recognition of the sedentary living pattern in this country. The calculation of protein needs was derived from the premise that the nitrogen requirement represents the sum of the losses of endogenous nitrogen in urine and feces, plus nitrogen in sweat, skin and other integumental losses. Reduction in the need for ascorbic acid was founded on recent studies with isotopes in presumably healthy men. Finally, the increase in iron requirements was based, in part, upon a recent study which indicated that iron stores were reduced or absent in two-thirds of menstruating women and the majority of pregnant women.

The RDA has proved useful in planning diets for population groups and as a standard of reference for dietary surveys of large samples. It is also a helpful method of comparing or establishing *average* requirements. However, the adequacy or inadequacy of the diets of individuals should not be judged on the basis of comparison with the RDA. In the final analysis, the disease problem at hand, as well as the results of clinical and biochemical appraisal of nutritional status, must be considered.

The Food and Nutrition Board recognizes that large segments of the population may benefit from dietary practices not specified in the RDA. For example, the Board acknowledges that reduction in serum cholesterol and triglyceride levels by dietary means would likely benefit "many Americans." But the Food and Nutrition Board maintains that this should be done on an individual basis. The Board further acknowledges that some authorities feel that diets high in sugars and saturated fats contribute to coronary heart disease and that "a diet high in sucrose may promote dental caries." Nevertheless, it does not make any recommendations regarding levels of intake for these nutrients. The American Medical Association urges physicians to make dietary recommendations, based upon clinical investigations, that go beyond the RDA to prevent as well as treat heart disease.

DAILY FOOD SELECTION

Three requirements are basic to the formulation of an optimal diet. First, it should be couched in terms readily grasped and understood by the general public. Few people will remember, much less consume for a protracted period, a diet in which precise portions (e.g., ounces, grams) of the various food groups are prescribed. Second, it must be economically realistic. Finally, the regime should avoid those foodstuffs which are reported to correlate with disease states and should encourage those which have been noted to enhance health. Probably the best that can be realistically achieved is an understanding of which foods are to be eaten liberally, sparingly, and to be avoided. It is the development of a rational life-long eating pattern rather than the following of a rigid diet that is to be encouraged.

Foods To Be Eaten Liberally: Many nutrients, when present in sufficient amounts, enhance the body's defenses against disease and when in short supply, decrease this defense. Such substances may be called *resistance* factors. These nutrients, which are well dispersed in a variety of foods, include protein, vitamins and minerals.

In a review of clinical nutrition studies (Diet and Disease—1968), these resistance nutrients were reported to affect favorably the body's defense against many allegedly nonnutritional disorders (infertility, obstetrical complications, congenital defects, mental retardation, psychologic disorders, cancer, and ischemic heart disease).

Protein, vitamins, and minerals, serving as resistance agents, throughout this book have been noted to produce more hope for the incurable.

The most nutritious protein foods, i.e., those containing all the essential amino acids in proper balance, are obtained largely from animal sources. Thus, animal protein is said to have high biologic value. Biologic value (BV) of protein is defined as the percentage of absorbed nitrogen retained in the body. The retention of nitrogen (i.e., protein) is equal to the ability of the protein to become tissue, since the body has little storage capacity with respect to protein. The fact that whole egg protein has a biologic value of 100 per cent means that it is able to replace, gram for gram, daily body losses of protein. The relative value of other proteins are: animal protein, 70 to 100; casein (milk protein), 70 to 75; wheat, 60; and vegetable protein, 40 to 65. Thus, besides making their own valuable contributions to the body's amino acid pool and protein stores, the presence of animal protein assures utilization of the amino acids from plant sources. For example, the amino acids amply provided by cereal foods cannot be used for the construction of a tissue protein unless the amino acid or acids lacking are supplied then and there from another source. Protein foods should be consumed in generous quantities at each meal. Excellent sources of animal protein, besides meat, fish and fowl, include eggs, hard cheeses and cottage cheese, and milk (including buttermilk and skim milk).

When available, one should eat daily fresh uncooked seasonal fruits. Ideally, one should be of the citrus variety. Raw fruits are preferable to those that have been cooked. If canned fruits must be consumed, the unsweetened forms are preferable. Fruit juices may be used in addition to fresh fruits and can serve as substitutes for soft drinks and other beverages. Any kind of fruit juice, canned, frozen, and fresh, except those with added sugar, is acceptable. The list of nutrient-rich vegetables is bountiful. The dark-green and deep-yellow varieties are excellent examples. These and others, such as the potato, should be consumed daily, both cooked and in the raw state. It is evident from the above description that the preferred foods are many and varied.

Foods to be Eaten Sparingly: There are foodstuffs which should be consumed in limited amounts because they have a relatively low essential nutrient-to-calorie ratio. Some of these foods are moderately priced. Therefore, they are useful in rounding out calorie requirements, especially when these are high. Such foods, in these circumstances, are said to have a protein-sparing effect since protein will simply be burned for energy if adequate fat and carbohydrate are not available to meet caloric requirements. However, as previously noted in the 1968 edition of the Recommended Dietary Allowances, the increasingly sedentary living pattern of this country suggests that there is more likelihood of the opposite problem, an excess of calories.

Breads and cereals (that require cooking) fit in this category. Within this group, the whole grain varieties are preferable. Saturated fats (e.g., fat on meats, butter and solid cooking fats) should be consumed sparingly and can be replaced with those of the unsaturated type (e.g., vegetable oil spreads and liquid cooking fats).

Artificial sweeteners should be used only in limited amounts. Caffeine-containing foods and drugs should be used sparingly. This is especially true in individuals who tend to have blood sugar values that are too high or too low. Examples of such foods and drugs are coffee, tea, cola drinks, Anacin, A.P.C., A.S.A. Compound, B.C., Caffergot, Coricidin, Empirin Compound, Fiorinal, Four Way Cold Tablets, Sulfayne, Stanback, and Trigesic.

Foods to be Avoided: Several nutrients, when consumed in relatively large quantities, increase the body's proneness to disease and, when limited, decrease its likelihood of becoming diseased. Such substances may be called *susceptibility* factors. These nutrients include the simple sugars (sucrose or table sugar), syrups, and the highly processed or refined starch foods.

Throughout this book, the restriction of highly processed carbohydrate foods (serving as a susceptibility agent) has been observed to produce more hope for the incurable.

It will be recalled that the major change in the American diet (Chapter Two) in the past eighty years has been a doubling of syrup and simple sugar consumption. This is noteworthy for four reasons.

First, sugar-rich foodstuffs, except for their caloric value, are nutrient-poor. Second, these nutrient-poor foods also require considerable quantities of vitamins and minerals for their metabolism. The potential body loss that can occur due to the tissue depleting action of these foods over a period of a year is surprising. Doctor Roth of New York City calculated this possible loss based on the 1930 per capita consumption of sugar which was 118 pounds.

1. 118 pounds of sugar per annum is equivalent to approximately 500 calories per day.
2. 500 calories of carbohydrate requires 0.25 mg. of thiamin and riboflavin among other enzymes and vitamins in order for the body to utilize the carbohydrates. Therefore, the body must obtain these nutrients from other foods since there is no storage of the water soluble vitamins in the body.
3. The deficit of Vitamins B_1 and B_2, besides many other important nutrients, may amount to 0.25 mg. per day each.
4. The deficit of thiamin and riboflavin alone could well be 90 mg. in a single year [$360 \times 0.25 = 90$].

The full significance of this loss becomes apparent when it is recalled that this is only an average figure for sugar consumption. Since many people consume little sugar, others must consume larger amounts. Such dietary patterns may persist for decades!

Third, these heavily sweetened foods frequently displace protein, vitamin and mineral-rich foodstuffs in the diet. It is interesting that the downward trend noted in American eating habits between 1955 and 1965 was ascribed to the decreased use of milk and milk products, fruits and vegetables, and a corresponding increase in the use of ready-baked goods.

Fourth, there are numerous reports which suggest that sugar may influence the incidence of clinically recognizable diabetes mellitus. It is estimated that more than one person in ten in the United States is either a known or unknown diabetic, a latent diabetic, or demonstrates an abnormal glucose tolerance. The link between diabetes mellitus and increased susceptibility to many chronic diseases (cancer, heart disease, gout, obesity, high blood pressure, pyorrhea, etc.) further underscores the significance of the high consumption trend.

In addition to the sugar naturally present in food, the following data (Dicalator Systems, Inc., 1957, P. O. Box 3217, Olympic Station, Beverly Hills, California) emphasize three facts regarding the simple sugars added to a variety of foods. First, some products are almost exclusively sugar (e.g., four ounces of hard candy contain 20 teaspoonsful). Second, sugar is frequently hidden in other foods (e.g., sweetened gelatin and canned fruits). Third, while certain products admittedly contain only small quantities of sugar (e.g., chewing gums and gum drops), the nature of their use makes for overall large sugar intake. In fact, simple sugars are added to a wide variety of processed foods (cereals, canned vegetables, and sauces).

HIDDEN SUGARS IN FOODS

The patient says, "Doc, I don't eat any sugar." Here are the approximate amounts of refined sugar (added sugar—in addition to the sugar naturally present) hidden in popular foods—about which the patient is usually unaware:

Food item	Size portion	Approximate sugar content in teaspoonsful of granulated sugar
BEVERAGES		
cola drinks	1 [6 oz. bottle or glass]	3½
cordials	1 [¾ oz. glass]	1½
gingerale	6 oz.	5

Food item	Size portion	Approximate sugar content in teaspoonsful of granulated sugar
hi-ball	1 [6 oz. glass]	2½
orange-ade	1 [8 oz. glass]	5
root beer	1 [10 oz. bottle]	4½
seven-up	1 [6 oz. bottle or glass]	3¾
soda pop	1 [8 oz. bottle]	5
sweet cider	1 cup	6
whiskey sour	1 [3 oz. glass]	1½
CAKES & COOKIES		
angel food	1 [4 oz. piece]	7
apple sauce cake	1 [4 oz. piece]	5½
banana cake	1 [2 oz. piece]	2
cheese cake	1 [4 oz. piece]	2
choc. cake [plain]	1 [4 oz. piece]	6
choc. cake [iced]	1 [4 oz. piece]	10
coffee cake	1 [4 oz. piece]	4½
cup cake [iced]	1	6
fruit cake	1 [4 oz. piece]	5
jelly roll	1 [2 oz. piece]	2½
orange cake	1 [4 oz. piece]	4
pound cake	1 [4 oz. piece]	5
sponge cake	1 [1 oz. piece]	2
strawberry shortcake	1 serving	4
brownies [unfrosted]	1 [¾ oz.]	3
chocolate cookies	1	1½
fig newtons	1	5
ginger snaps	1	3
macaroons	1	6
nut cookies	1	1½
oatmeal cookies	1	2
sugar cookies	1	1½

Food item	Size portion	Approximate sugar content in teaspoonsful of granulated sugar
chocolate eclair	1	7
cream puff	1	2
donut [plain]	1	3
donut [glazed]	1	6
snail	1 [4 oz. piece]	4½

CANDIES

average choc. milk bar	1 [1½ oz.]	2½
chewing gum	1 stick	½
chocolate cream	1 piece	2
butterscotch chew	1 piece	1
chocolate mints	1 piece	2
fudge	1 oz. square	4½
gumdrop	1	2
hard candy	4 oz.	20
lifesavers	1	⅓
peanut brittle	1 oz.	3½

CANNED FRUITS & JUICES

canned apricots	4 halves & 1 Tb. syrup	3½
canned fruit juices [sweet]	½ cup	2
canned peaches	2 halves & 1 Tb. syrup	3½
fruit salad	½ cup	3½
fruit syrup	2 Tb.	2½
stewed fruits	½ cup	2

DAIRY PRODUCTS

ice cream	⅓ pt. [3½ oz.]	3½
ice cream bar	1	1-7 depending on size
ice cream cone	1	3½
ice cream soda	1	5
ice cream sundae	1	7
malted milk shake	1 [10 oz. glass]	5

Food item	Size portion	Approximate sugar content in teaspoonsful of granulated sugar
JAMS & JELLIES		
apple butter	1 Tb.	1
jelly	1 Tb.	4-6
orange marmalade	1 Tb.	4-6
peach butter	1 Tb.	1
strawberry jam	1 Tb.	4
DESSERTS, MISCELLANEOUS		
apple cobbler	½ cup	3
blueberry cobbler	½ cup	3
custard	½ cup	2
french pastry	1 [4 oz. piece]	5
jello	½ cup	4½
apple pie	1 slice [average]	7
apricot pie	1 slice	7
berry pie	1 slice	10
butterscotch pie	1 slice	4
cherry pie	1 slice	10
cream pie	1 slice	4
lemon pie	1 slice	7
mince meat pie	1 slice	4
peach pie	1 slice	7
prune pie	1 slice	6
pumpkin pie	1 slice	5
rhubarb pie	1 slice	4
banana pudding	½ cup	2
bread pudding	½ cup	1½
chocolate pudding	½ cup	4
cornstarch pudding	½ cup	2½
date pudding	½ cup	7
fig pudding	½ cup	7
grapenut pudding	½ cup	2
plum pudding	½ cup	4
rice pudding	½ cup	5
tapioca pudding	½ cup	3
berry tart	½ cup	10

Food item	Size portion	Approximate sugar content in teaspoonsful of granulated sugar
blanc mange	½ cup	5
brown betty	½ cup	3
plain pastry	1 [4 oz. piece]	3
sherbet	½ cup	9

SYRUP, SUGARS & ICINGS

Food item	Size portion	Approximate sugar content in teaspoonsful of granulated sugar
brown sugar	1 Tb.	3 [actual sugar content]
chocolate icing	1 oz.	5
chocolate sauce	1 Tb.	3½
corn syrup	1 Tb.	3 [actual sugar content]
granulated sugar	1 Tb.	3 [actual sugar content]
honey	1 Tb.	3 [actual sugar content]
karo syrups	1 Tb.	3 [actual sugar content]
maple syrup	1 Tb.	5 [actual sugar content]
molasses	1 Tb.	3½ [actual sugar content]
white icing	1 oz.	5

The avoidance of such foods in our present culture is extremely difficult. Sweets are the foods commonly consumed because of their reward and snack appeal. In their stead, tissue-building foods rich in protein, minerals, and vitamins are indicated. Fruits, fruit juices, nuts, cheeses, and raw vegetables serve as desirable snack or dessert substitutes. Adequate nutrient intake, especially protein, at mealtimes mutes the desire for between-meal sweets.

Economic Aspects: Dietary selection is, in part, economically determined. Table 1 portrays the marked variation
in nutrients furnished per ten cents' worth of soft drinks and
fruit juices. It is evident that the soft drinks contain only
carbohydrates and calories. In contrast, the juices include an
array of vital nutrients. Table 2 similarly reveals comparative
cost and quality (plant versus animal source) of protein furnished by representative foods frequently purchased for household consumption. For the same dollar, it is possible to obtain
food rich or poor in nourishment. On this basis, some *economy*
foods (e.g., cornflakes) are actually exorbitantly priced.

TABLE 1

Comparison of nutrients furnished per ten cents'
worth of soft drinks and fruit juices

Nutrients	Tomato juice [12 oz.]	Orange juice [4 oz. frozen]	Grape fruit juice [4 oz. frozen]	Ginger ale [8 oz.]	Cola drinks [8 oz.]
protein [gm.]	3.6	0.4	0.3	0	0
fat [gm.]	0.7	1.0	0.5	0	0
carbohydrate [gm.]	15.0	50.0	52.0	20	19
calories	75.0	200.0	200.0	86	78
calcium [mg.]	25.0	46.0	42.0	0	0
phosphorus [mg.]	54.0	80.0	68.0	0	0
iron [mg.]	1.5	1.4	1.6	0	0
Vitamin A [I.U.]	3800.0	440.0	40.0	0	0
thiamin [mg.]	0.2	0.3	0.2	0	0
riboflavin [mg.]	0.1	0.1	0.1	0	0
nicotinic acid [mg.]	2.7	1.0	1.0	0	0
ascorbic acid [mg.]	60.0	180.0	180.0	0	0

TABLE 2

Comparative cost and quality [*plant versus animal source*]
of protein furnished by representative foods

Foods	Cost per* pound	Grams protein** pound	Cost of 100 grams protein
Plant sources			
oatmeal	0.30	64	0.47
sugar-covered cornflakes	0.40	20	2.00
white, enriched bread, 4% milk solids	0.20	40	0.50
whole wheat bread, 2% milk solids	0.24	48	0.50
Animal sources [meat]			
beef sirloin	1.29	71	1.82
frankfurters, all meat	0.65	59	1.10
ground meat, regular	0.56	81	0.69
Animal sources [dairy]			
whole milk 3.5% fat	0.15	16	0.94
ice cream	0.30	18	1.67
powdered skim [non-fat solids] instant	0.46	162	0.28

Nutrient-Calorie Relationships: Breakfast, lunch, and dinner menus which make every calorie count, nutrientwise, are compared with inadequate, isocaloric (same number of calories) meals in Tables 3, 4, and 5. It becomes quite evident that the caloric yield in terms of tissue building nutrients can be markedly increased through wise food selection. The Recommended Dietary Allowances proposed by the Food and Nutrition Board of the National Research Council for most Americans (RDA, 7th Revised Edition, 1968) leaves little room for nutrient-poor foods. Thus, the prime need in dietary guidance is to make the patient aware of the relative nutrient value of foods. These have been extensively reviewed and

*Supermarket prices. 18 February 1969.
**Protein content on basis of Agriculture Handbook No. 8 U.S. Dept. of Agriculture, 1963.

published by the United States Department of Agriculture (Composition of Foods, Raw, Processed, Prepared, Handbook No. 8).

Snacks: Between-meal eating is not necessarily an undesirable habit. In fact, evidence suggests that spreading the daily food intake over five or six meals, without increasing the total amount, is desirable. It has been reported to stabilize blood sugar levels, decrease fatigue and prevent obesity.

The selection of the foods eaten at these between-meal "meals" is important. They should be chosen from the *Foods To Be Eaten Liberally* rather than the *Foods To Be Eaten Sparingly* or *Avoided* groups. Unfortunately, the temptation is to eat foods from these last two groups because they are usually more readily available. Resist this temptation!

TABLE 3

Comparative nutritional value of two isocaloric breakfasts

Nutrients	Adequate* breakfast [700 calories]	Inadequate** breakfast [700 calories]	Adequate: inadequate ratio
ascorbic acid [mg.]	50	0.0	50.0
nicotinic acid [mg.]	15	0.6	25.0
phosphorus [mg.]	760	100	7.6
calcium [mg.]	460	65	7.1
riboflavin [mg.]	1.07	0.18	5.9
protein [gram]	45	8	5.6
iodine [mcg.]	17	4	4.3
iron [mg.]	7	2	3.5
Vitamin A [I.U.]	4200	1400	3.0
thiamin [mg.]	0.8	0.4	2.0
fat [gram]	40	30	1.3
carbohydrate [gram]	40	100	0.4

*½ grapefruit, 2 eggs, 3 oz. ham. 1 slice whole grain bread and butter, 1 glass of milk.

**3 hot cakes with butter and syrup, 1 cup coffee with sugar and cream.

TABLE 4

Comparative nutritional value of two isocaloric lunches

Nutrients	Adequate* lunch [655 calories]	Inadequate** lunch [655 calories]	Adequate: inadequate ratio
iodine [mcg.]	34	1.4	24.3
ascorbic acid [mg.]	10	1	10.0
iron [mg.]	4	0.6	6.7
riboflavin [mg.]	0.53	0.1	5.3
calcium [mg.]	370	75	4.9
Vitamin A [I.U.]	1930	420	4.6
phosphorus [mg.]	440	120	3.7
thiamin [mg.]	0.26	0.07	3.7
protein [gram]	28	11	2.5
fat [gram]	27	21	1.3
nicotinic acid [mg.]	3	2.5	1.2
carbohydrate [gram]	75	105	0.7

*1 bowl vegetable soup, shrimp salad, 1 slice whole grain bread and butter, 1 glass buttermilk, 1 apple.

**1 ham sandwich, 1 soft drink, 1 piece of pie.

TABLE 5

Comparative nutritional value of two isocaloric dinners

Nutrients	Adequate* dinner [890 calories]	Inadequate** dinner [890 calories]	Adequate: inadequate ratio
ascorbic acid [mg.]	90	10	9.0
riboflavin [mg.]	1.4	0.29	4.8
iodine [mcg.]	45	11	4.1
nicotinic acid [mg.]	16	4.5	3.6
calcium [mg.]	600	175	3.4
thiamin [mg.]	0.84	0.26	3.2
phosphorus [mg.]	860	321	2.7
Vitamin A [I.U.]	4900	1900	2.6
protein [gram]	70	28	2.5
iron [mg.]	10	4	2.5
fat [gram]	30	40	0.8
carbohydrate [gram]	85	105	0.8

*4 oz. tomato juice, mixed green salad with vinegar dressing, 6 oz. roast beef, baked potato with 1 square butter, green peas, ½ canteloupe with 1 oz. cheddar cheese, 1 glass buttermilk.

**Spaghetti and meat balls, mixed salad with french dressing, french bread and 1 square butter, french pastry, coffee with sugar and cream.

DINING ENVIRONMENT

Colorless, drab or tasteless meals, no matter how nutritious, are of little value if not eaten, or if eaten but not assimilated. Appetite and the flow of digestive juices can be greatly stimulated or depressed by the appearance, aroma and flavor of foods.

Equally important are the surroundings and circumstances under which food is consumed. Family arguments, noise, melodramatic TV programs—any stimulus which excites the primeval *fight or flight* reaction of man—not only works against food assimilation but actively promotes the development of gastrointestinal disturbances. In contrast, relaxed conversation or soft music contribute substantially to good, healthy digestion. These aspects of diet receive far too little emphasis.

DIETARY SUPPLEMENTATION

Because of the severe nutrient loss from foods (Chapter Three) between the garden and the gullet (via transportation, storage, processing, freezing, thawing, rinsing, cooking, after-cooking time lapse, and many others), it is quite unlikely that the RDA for all nutrients can be obtained from food alone. Even the consumption of an optimal diet as just presented is no assurance of an optimal nutrient intake.

Absorption, utilization and requirements for vitamins, minerals, protein and other important nutrients are all quite individually tailored. For many of the essential nutrients there are differences in individual requirements, ranging from two to ten fold. It has been shown, for instance, that in healthy young men of the same racial stock, a 4.5 range exists in individual calcium requirements. For particular amino acids (the building blocks of protein), one presumably healthy person may require 6.5 times as much as another. In experimental lower animals, even within a given strain, there may be as much as a 25-fold difference in requirements.

Actually, for a given nutrient there is no set amount that will serve everyone. For this reason, perfectly safe nutrients should be taken in excess of the average need as insurance against possible deficiency.

Suboptimal Dietary Intake: Many people find it difficult to maintain an optimum dietary intake. It may well be that those in this category contribute significantly to the increasing number of Americans, 50 per cent in 1965 as opposed to 40 per cent in 1955, who fail to eat an adequate diet (Chapter Three). Occupations requiring extensive traveling, irregular hours, or frequent entertaining may create such a situation. The executive fits this category. The nutritional dilemma of such an individual has been described and studied by investigators at the Research Institute of the Hospital for Sick Children, Toronto. Typically, he may have a martini at lunch and before dinner, wine with dinner, liqueur with coffee and whiskey for a nightcap. This *hypothetical 70 kg. sedentary individual is obtaining almost half of his recommended 2,400 calories daily through alcohol and other empty calories.*

There are other individuals who are limited in the variety of foods they eat. Included under this heading would be persons with very restricted food preferences, those subject to food allergies or incompatibilities, people suffering from lack of appetite, and patients on therapeutic diets (e.g., the Sippy diet for gastritis and peptic ulcer). Still another group are those with various emotional or behavioral problems. The psychologically disturbed, the heavy social drinker, the alcoholic, those who crave sweets (during an emotional crisis or hypoglycemic period), and those whose smoking impairs the appetite or who turn to snacks as a substitute for smoking, are typical of this segment of the population.

There are people with religious, social, or cultural taboos which make consumption of an optimum diet difficult. For example, vegetarians may find it hard to achieve the desired intake of high quality protein. Finally, there are many individuals who have poor dietary habits, and are aware of the fact but have no wish or intention of changing. Such people are frequently willing to take supplements if this will partially compensate for their poor dietary habits.

It is extremely important that patients not acquire the illusion that poor dietary habits can be completely offset by vitamin and mineral supplementation. It should be made clear to them that supplements in lieu of an optimum diet are, at best, a poor compromise and a crutch of limited value. They should be made to understand, for example, that vitamin and mineral formulations may not be as effectively assimilated as the nutrients in foodstuffs. They also cannot substitute for inadequate protein or unsaturated fat intake; nor can they counter many of the undesirable effects of a high sugar intake, or obviate the problems of excess calorie consumption. Yet to deny them the benefits of at least partial correction of their malnutrition would seem illogical.

Iron Requirements: Special mention should be made of the problem of iron intake. An important change in the 1968 RDA is the increase to 18 mg. daily for females from the age of ten years to menopause. This was based to some extent on a recent study which indicated that iron stores were reduced or absent in two-thirds of menstruating, and the majority of pregnant women.

Dietary surveys suggest that ordinary mixed diets provide about 5 to 6 mg. of iron for every 1,000 calories. Thus, girls and women consuming 2,000 calories or less daily find it difficult to obtain more than 10 to 12 mg. of iron per day. Even 18 mg. of iron daily do not meet the requirements of women with abnormally large menstrual losses, or during pregnancy. Such individuals may require as much as two and one-half times this amount of iron. This requirement cannot be derived from diet and should be met by iron supplementation. Although the prescription of iron during pregnancy is increasingly common, it is not yet routine.

Digestants: In the opinion of some authorities, malfunction of the digestive processes may require not only nutrient supplementation but the addition of one or more of the digestive secretions. In one study of 3,484 persons selected because of their complaints of oral and gastrointestinal distress, 27 per cent were found to have achlorhydria (little or no stomach acid) with an increasing frequency in the aged. It is thought that these individuals may not be able to assimilate or retain a sufficient amount of proper nutritive substances from even the most carefully directed diets. Hydrochloric acid, vitamin and mineral supplementation is essential for the proper assimilation of food. Bile salts may be needed after cholecystectomy (gall bladder removal). Pancreatin may be prescribed when nutrition is a problem in chronic pancreatitis.

Dietary Supplements: Due to the complexity of body processes and the dynamics of nutrient interrelationships, nutritional therapy will always remain, in some measure, an art as well as a science. However, there are several principles which should serve as guidelines in the use of supplements.

First, vitamin and mineral supplements *cannot* take the place of proper daily food selection. Supplements in lieu of an optimum diet are, at best, a crutch of limited value.

Second, although single nutrients can be beneficial, it has been clearly established that deficiencies of single nutrients rarely, if ever, occur. Further, nutrient interrelationships are extremely complex. Lack of one can affect the requirements for another. Thus, the prescription of multiple nutrients is the method of choice.

Third, as a basic supplement, the most desirable one is a formula that is complete in terms of essential nutrients present in dosage levels sufficient to meet all of the body's needs.

Fourth, harmful effects from overdosage are rarely encountered, and these have been almost exclusively in extremely high dosage levels of Vitamins A and D, for example, given separately. Early symptoms of toxicity have not been observed in adults except in dosage levels of at least 50,000 units daily of Vitamin D for several weeks, and dangerous calcification of the renal parenchyma occurs only when doses are as high as 300,000-500,000 units daily for long periods. Ingestion of several million units are required to produce hypervitaminosis A; excessive doses ingested over six months or longer usually antedate clinical manifestations as reported in the literature. Nicotinic acid may cause a vasodilator action, characterized by flushing and itching; but, in fact, this action is exploited in the treatment of conditions benefited by vasodilatation. This effect is avoided in most vitamin formulas by substituting nicotinamide for nicotinic acid. A few cases of sensitization to thiamin have been reported following repeated injections.

Fifth, when increased stress is anticipated, higher dosage levels should be given.

Sixth, in view of the wide margin of safety in dosage levels, the broad variation in nutrient requirements in different patients and in the same patient at different times and the relatively modest cost of supplements (as compared to candy, soft drinks, cigarettes, and liquor, for example), it is wiser to overdose (the only consequence being excretion of the unused nutrients, especially in the case of nutrients other than Vitamins A and D) than risk not meeting nutrient needs. Parenthetic mention should be made that even excreted nutrients may be beneficial. One and a half grams (1500 mg.) of ascorbic acid daily has been prescribed by Doctor Jorgen V. Schlegel, Chairman of Tulane University's Urology Department, to prevent recurrences of carcinoma of the urinary bladder according to a recent report to the American Association of Genito-Urinary Surgeons. This level of intake assures spillage into the urine. The presence of the ascorbate in the urine appears to prevent the formation of carcinogenic metabolites.

Seventh, a basic vitamin-mineral supplement may need reinforcement by more specialized formulas to meet specific needs. A *stress* water-soluble vitamin formula may be indicated prior to surgery. Increased amounts of bioflavonoids and ascorbic acid may be indicated in patients with persistent indications of capillary fragility, bleeding, and/or suboptimal tissue levels of vitamin C. Persons with histories of excessive, recurrent blood loss, women with heavy menstrual flow, and marginal red blood cell levels when pregnant may benefit from an iron formula. On the basis of recent clinical findings, 500 mg. of ascorbic acid daily may be desirable initially to prevent the formation of tartar on the teeth. Finally, the need for calcium by the teenage female, for those pregnant, and for the prevention of osteoporosis (bone thinning) must be met with additional supplementation.

Many other examples of the need for specialized formulas to reinforce a basic vitamin-mineral supplement could be cited. A doctor who is knowledgeable about diet and nutrition is aware of these additional requirements.

General Information About Supplements: Two basic formulas provide the patterns for most vitamin and vitamin-mineral preparations. Vitamin supplementation at a level of about one-third to twice the RDA has been suggested as a means of maintaining normal tissue reserves against the demands of illness, injury, pregnancy, or other unusual stress situations in individuals already in an optimal nutritional state. Such formulas are called *supplemental* or *maintenance* preparations. The pregnancy or prenatal variations of this formula usually contain Vitamin K and more calcium and more Vitamin B₆.

When individuals are in varying degrees of suboptimal nutriture, *therapeutic* preparations are prescribed. These contain from two to ten times the RDA for the various vitamins. "T" when present in the name of a preparation usually indicates that the vitamin fractions are present in therapeutic amounts. A variation in the *therapeutic* formula omits the fat-soluble vitamins (A, D, and E). The hypothetical basis for this variation, called a *stress* formula, is that the body stores the fat-soluble vitamins and hence they are not as likely to become depleted in stressful situations. *Stress* formulas differ from *supplemental* and regular *therapeutic* formulas also in that they may contain larger quantities of Vitamin C and digestive enzymes.

It needs to be underscored that the terms *supplemental, maintenance, therapeutic,* or *stress* relate only to the vitamin content of such formulas and not to the minerals if these are included in the preparation. Almost all of multivitamin formulations contain all or at least most of the vitamin fractions for which allowances were established in the 1963 RDA. Most contain the vitamin fractions or a large portion of those for which allowances were established in the 1968 RDA. Some contain those considered as essential but for which no RDA is established (Vitamin K, inositol, choline, biotin, pantothenic acid, and bioflavonoids).

The addition of minerals to a multivitamin preparation usually increases the price only slightly. The amount of mineral present in the *therapeutic* formulas is not necessarily greater than the amounts in the *supplemental* formulas. In neither formula do the amounts of minerals approach the RDA levels except in the case of iron, iodine, and copper.

Representative formulas usually contain from two-thirds to twice the RDA for iron and iodine, from one-sixteenth to one-third that for calcium and phosphorus, and about one per cent of the RDA for magnesium. These are the only ones for which allowances have been established. Others commonly added to formulas and the per cent of their estimated daily need are zinc (5 to 10 per cent), copper (50 to 100 per cent), potassium (0 to 0.5 per cent), and manganese (12 to 33 per cent). Still others which are regarded as essential but which are seldom present in formulas are chromium, molybdenum, and selenium.

Desiccated liver and/or brewer's yeast may be provided as additional supplements. These foods are not only excellent sources of the B-complex vitamins and other known nutritional factors but are good protein supplements as well. Digestive enzymes are occasionally provided to aid the absorption and utilization of all nutrients. Biotin, choline, inositol, and lecithin are sometimes used to aid lipid metabolism.

All nutritional supplements are more effectively utilized when taken with meals and when provided more than once daily.

SUMMARY

Certain nutrients in the diet increase the body's defenses against disease when present in sufficient amounts and decrease this defense when in short supply. These nutrients, protein, vitamins and minerals, may be termed *resistance* factors.

Other nutrients, when consumed in large quantities, increase the body's proneness to disease, and, when restricted, decrease its likelihood of becoming diseased. These nutrients, primarily table sugar and highly processed (refined) carbohydrate (starch), may be called *susceptibility* factors.

Thus, the consumption of *resistance* nutrients is to be encouraged but intake of the *susceptibility* nutrients should be restricted.

It is unlikely that an individual's nutrient needs or requirements can be achieved with food alone. For this reason, and many others, nutrients should be taken in excess of the average need as insurance against possible deficiency.

For guidance concerning diet and dietary supplements, consult a doctor knowledgeable about these dynamic preventive tools.

RECOMMENDED DAILY ALLOWANCES FOR CALORIES
AND PROTEIN FOR AGES 10 TO 75 +
[*Food and Nutrition Board of the National
Research Council, Revised 1968*]

	Age* *years from up to*	*Weight* *kg.*	*[lbs]*	*Height* *cm*	*[in]*	*Cal- ories*	*Protein* *gm*
Males	10-12	35	77	140	55	2500	45
	12-14	43	95	151	59	2700	50
	14-18	59	130	170	67	3000	60
	18-22	67	147	175	69	2800	60
	22-35	70	154	175	69	2800	65
	35-55	70	154	173	68	2600	65
	55-75+	70	154	171	67	2400	65
Females	10-12	35	77	142	56	2250	50
	12-14	44	97	154	61	2300	50
	14-16	52	114	157	62	2400	55
	16-18	54	119	160	63	2300	55
	18-22	58	128	163	64	2000	55
	22-35	58	128	163	64	2000	55
	35-55	58	128	160	63	1850	55
	55-75+	58	128	157	62	1700	55
Pregnancy						+200	65
Lactation						+1000	75

*Entries on lines for age-range 22-35 years represent the reference man and woman at age 22. All other entries represent allowances for the midpoint of the specified age range.

RECOMMENDED DAILY ALLOWANCES FOR

FAT SOLUBLE VITAMINS, AGE 10 TO 75+

[*Food and Nutrition Board of the National*

Research Council, revised 1968]

	Age years from up to	Vitamin A activity I.U.	Vitamin D I.U.	Vitamin E activity I.U.
Males	10-12	4500	400	20
	12-14	5000	400	20
	14-18	5000	400	25
	18-22	5000	400	30
	22-35	5000	—	30
	35-55	5000	—	30
	55-75+	5000	—	30
Females	10-12	4500	400	20
	12-14	5000	400	20
	14-16	5000	400	25
	16-18	5000	400	25
	18-22	5000	400	25
	22-35	5000	—	25
	35-55	5000	—	25
	55-75+	5000	—	25
Pregnancy		6000	400	30
Lactation		8000	400	30

RECOMMENDED DAILY ALLOWANCES FOR
WATER SOLUBLE VITAMINS, AGES 10 TO 75+
[*Food and Nutrition Board of the National
Research Council, revised 1968*]

	Age years from up to	Ascorbic Acid mg	Fol-acin* mg	Niacin mg equiv.**	Ribo-flavin mg	Thia-mine mg	Vita-min B_6 mg	Vita-min B_{12} ug
Males	10-12	40	0.4	17	1.3	1.3	1.4	5
	12-14	45	0.4	18	1.4	1.4	1.6	5
	14-18	55	0.4	20	1.5	1.5	1.8	5
	18-22	60	0.4	18	1.6	1.4	2.0	5
	22-35	60	0.4	18	1.7	1.4	2.0	5
	35-55	60	0.4	17	1.7	1.3	2.0	5
	55-75+	60	0.4	14	1.7	1.2	2.0	6
Females	10-12	40	0.4	15	1.3	1.1	1.4	5
	12-14	45	0.4	15	1.4	1.2	1.6	5
	14-16	50	0.4	16	1.4	1.2	1.8	5
	16-18	50	0.4	15	1.5	1.2	2.0	5
	18-22	55	0.4	13	1.5	1.0	2.0	5
	22-35	55	0.4	13	1.5	1.0	2.0	5
	35-55	55	0.4	13	1.5	1.0	2.0	5
	55-75+	55	0.4	13	1.5	1.0	2.0	6
Pregnancy		60	0.8	15	1.8	+0.1	2.5	8
Lactation		60	0.5	20	2.0	+0.5	2.5	6

*The folacin allowances refer to dietary sources as determined by Lactobacillus casei assay. Pure forms of folacin may be effective in doses less than ¼ of the RDA.

**Niacin equivalents include dietary sources of the vitamin itself plus 1 mg equivalent for each 60 mg of dietary tryptophan.

RECOMMENDED DIETARY ALLOWANCES
FOR MINERALS, AGES 10 TO 75+
*[Food and Nutrition Board of the National
Research Council, revised 1968]*

	Age years from up to	Calcium gm	Phos- phorus gm	Iodine ug	Iron mg	Mag- nesium mg
Males	10-12	1.2	1.2	125	10	300
	12-14	1.4	1.4	135	18	350
	14-18	1.4	1.4	150	18	400
	18-22	0.8	0.8	140	10	400
	22-35	0.8	0.8	140	10	350
	35-55	0.8	0.8	125	10	350
	55-75+	0.8	0.8	110	10	350
Females	10-12	1.2	1.2	110	18	300
	12-14	1.3	1.3	115	18	350
	14-16	1.3	1.3	120	18	350
	16-18	1.3	1.3	115	18	350
	18-22	0.8	0.8	100	18	350
	22-35	0.8	0.8	100	18	300
	35-55	0.8	0.8	90	18	300
	55-75+	0.8	0.8	80	10	300
Pregnancy		+0.4	+0.4	125	18	450
Lactation		+0.5	+0.5	150	18	450

IMPORTANT REVISION IN THE 1968
RECOMMENDED DIETARY ALLOWANCES
[RDA], ages 10 to 75+, as compared to the 1964 revision

Nutrients added for which specific allowances established

	Male	Female
Vitamin E [I.U.]	30.0	25.0
Folacin [mg.]	0.4	0.4
Vitamin B₆ [mg.]	2.0	2.0
Magnesium [mg.]	350.0	300.0
Phosphorus [gm.]	0.8	0.8
Iodine [mcg.]	110-140	80-100

	Male	*Female*
Requirements lowered	*1968*	*1964*
Calories, reference man	2800	2900
reference woman	2000	2100
Protein, reference man	65 gm.	70 gm.
reference woman	55 gm.	58 gm.
Ascorbic acid, adult males	60 mg.	70 mg.
adult females	55 mg.	70 mg.

Requirements increased

Iron, menstruating and pregnant females	18 mg.	15 mg.

REFERENCES

1. *Alcoholism a diet problem?* Rodale's Health Bulletin 5: #17, 9, 29 April 1967.
2. *Ascorbic acid regimen may induce calculus.* Dental Times 11: #12, 1, 15 December 1968.
3. Cheraskin, E. Ringsdorf, W. M., Jr., and Clark, J. W. *Diet and disease.* 1968. Emmaus, Pennsylvania, Rodale Books.
4. Consumer and Food Economics Research Division, Agriculture Research Service, United States Department of Agriculture. *Composition of foods, raw, processed, prepared,* Agriculture Handbook No. 8. Washington, D.C., United States Government Printing Office, December 1963.
5. *Dietary levels of households in the United States, Spring, 1965; a preliminary report.* ARS 62-17. United States Department of Agriculture Research Service, January 1968.
6. Editorial. *Nutritional requirements held unpredictable.* Geriatric Focus 9: #2, February 1970.
7. Food and Nutrition Board. *Recommended dietary allowances.* Seventh revised edition. 1968. Washington, D.C., National Academy of Sciences, National Research Council. Publication #1694.
8. Goodhart, R. S. *The diagnosis and management of malnutrition.* Medical Clinics of North America 45: #6, 1533-1540, November 1961.

9. Hodges, R. E. *Present knowledge of nutrition in relation to diabetes mellitus.* Chapter IX. *Present knowledge in nutrition.* 1967. New York, Nutrition Foundation, Inc.

10. Lyght, C. E., editor. *The Merck manual of diagnosis and therapy.* 1966. Eleventh edition. Rahway, New Jersey, Merck and Company, Inc.

11. *Minimum daily requirements.* Washington, D.C., United States Food and Drug Administration, Federal Food, Drug and Cosmetic Act, Section 403, Federal Register, 1 June 1951.

12. Nizel, A. E. *The science of nutrition and its application in clinical dentistry.* 1966. Second edition. Philadelphia, W. B. Saunders Company.

13. *Nutrition pot-pourri.* Food and Nutrition News 39: #7, 2, April 1968.

14. Orent-Keiles, E. and Hallman, L. F. *The breakfast meal in relation to blood sugar values.* Circular No. 827. Washington, D.C., United States Department of Agriculture, December 1949.

15. Pritchard, J. A. and Mason, R. A. *Iron stores of normal adults and replenishment with oral iron therapy.* Journal of the American Medical Association 190: #10, 879-901, 7 December 1964.

16. Robinson, C. H. *Planning the high protein diet.* In Practical diet therapy. Reprinted from American Journal of Clinical Nutrition 1955.

17. *Roth, H. The role of nutrition in periodontal and oral health.* New York State Dental Journal 26: #10, 459-468, December 1960.

18. Sharp, G. S. and Fister, H. W. *The diagnosis and treatment of achlorhydria: a ten year study.* Journal of the American Geriatric Society 15: #8, 786-791, August 1967.

19. Stahl, S. S. *The etiology of periodontal disease—review of literature.* World Workshop in Periodontics. 1966. Ann Arbor, University of Michigan Press, pp. 129-177.

20. Stanton, G. *The relation of diet to salivary calculus formation.* Journal of Periodontics-Periodontology 40: #3, 167-172, March 1967.

21. The Upjohn Company. *Vitamin manual; a Scope Monograph.* Kalamazoo, Michigan, 1965.

22. Walsh, M. J. *Nutrition by the calorie and by the dollar.* 1954. Beverly Hills, California.

23. White, H. S. *The critical question of dietary iron.* Food and Nutrition News 39: #7, 1, April 1968.

24. White, P. L. *Diet and the possible prevention of coronary atheroma; a Council on Foods and Nutrition statement.* Journal of the American Medical Association 194: #10, 1149-1150, 6 December 1965.